Hair Loss

Ultimate Guide To Learn About Hair Loss Prevention Methods And Regrowth Treatment

(Natural Hair Growth Secrets & Hair Loss Cure)

Clark Ranfield

Published By **Darby Connor**

Clark Ranfield

Hair Loss: Ultimate Guide To Learn About Hair Loss Prevention Methods And Regrowth Treatment (Natural Hair Growth Secrets & Hair Loss Cure)

ISBN   978-1-77485-978-0

Legal & Disclaimer

Table Of Contents

Chapter 1: How to Lose Hair

Hair grows all over the body. Hair is found everywhere, apart from our palms and our soles. Keratin is the protein our body uses to grow hair. The old hair cells are being pushed out of the skin's outer layer, which is what we perceive as hair. The hairs we see are actually made of strings of old, dead keratin cell strings. Science has shown that our hair grows on average six inches per annum.

It is so annoying that every time you go to take a shower, the floor of your bathroom is covered in fallen hairs. When you are just casually combing your hair and notice how many hairs are stuck in its teeth when you look at it. When your hair is not growing as fast or as thickly as it used to?

Studies have shown that hair loss is more common in males than in women. Male pattern baldness accounts for most of these cases. But, it is not uncommon for women to lose or thinning their hair. It is why so many cosmetic products claim to combat hair loss. This is not only common for women, but also demoralizing.

True, it is true that people today are obsessed with looking good, especially for women. The best way to reflect the beauty they have is through their hair. For many, having beautiful hair is an important part of their beauty. Researchers have found that women who experience hair loss or thinning hair are more likely to feel insecure and to have lower self-esteem. They may feel embarrassed about their condition.

Although hair loss is common and easy to treat, it can also be caused by many factors. To find the best solution, you must identify the cause. Male pattern hair loss is a leading reason that many men lose their hair as early as they are teenagers. This is a hereditary problem in men that results in a receding or thinned head.

Androgenic alopecia is the scientific term for Male Pattern Baldness. This is more common among men than in women. This condition can strike males in their teens and early twenties. However, this condition can lead to noticeable thinning of the hair in women who are already in their 40s. Males who suffer from this condition may experience a slow disappearance in their hair from their crown to their frontal area, while females might notice noticeable thinning around their crowns.

What is causing male pattern baldness in nearly 80% of the world? Scientists and researchers agree that this phenomenon may be caused by a substance in our bodies that circulates through the body. This substance, dihydrotestosterone is also known as DHT. This is what causes hair follicles in our hair to shrink and lay dormant.

Study results show that DHT is produced by converting testosterone into it through an enzyme known as 5a-reductase. These studies show that 5areductase has two types: Type 1 and 2. Type 1 contains only one-third, while Type 2 has two-thirds of the total DHT found in our bodies. Type 1 is found in the sebaceous cells of the skin, which includes our hair. Type 2 5a–reductase enzyme can be found at our hair's follicles.

Research has shown that males suffering from male pattern hair loss are more likely than others to have small hair roots and higher levels of DHT. Researchers have also shown that males with 5a reductase deficiency are not affected by Male Pattern Hair Loss.

It is exhausting though. This is just the tip. Other than the hormones & enzymes being circulated within our body, and the inherited genes that our parents gave us, there are many more external factors that may affect our health that we don't even know about. Some of these factors may be in our lives, others may be in the surroundings we live. It doesn't matter how minor or major, any factor can cause hair loss. This list contains the causes of hair fall and how to treat it.

Physical Stress

Hair loss can result from any type of trauma such as surgery, accident, or severe illness. This is known as Telogen Effluvium. Marc Glashofer, a New York City-based dermatologist, said that this condition affects three stages of the hair's natural life cycle. The growth stage is the first. Next comes the rest phase. And then the final stage is the shedding stage. He explained that your hair may become irritated by an event or trauma, and this could cause your hair to go into the shedding phase. A study showed that hair loss can begin three to six years after the event. Good news is that hair will start growing back once your body has recovered. Your hair will grow back quicker if you heal quickly.

Pulled-back Hair

This is quite common among women, but men are becoming more conscious of the importance of long hair. Do not wear your hair in tight braids, like dreadlocks. This can impact the growth of your hair. Also, hair can fall if it is pulled back too tightly like a ponytail. This is called traction alopecia. Because the hair is being pulled constantly, it can cause gradual hair loss.

Pregnancy

This is not true for men. Hair loss may be a result of pregnancy. This kind of hair fall is more common after you have given birth than during pregnancy. This is a common problem for women. Your hair will grow back in a few weeks.

Too Much Vitamin A

This is a testimony to the saying, "Too many is not good". Vitamin A gives the body essentials like better vision. But, as with all substances, excess Vitamin A is bad for your body. The American Academy of Dermatology suggests that we should get 5,000 International Units of Vitamin A each day for adults. Supplements for children aged four and over can contain as many as 2,500 to 10,000IU. This is a treatable condition. When your body has used up all of the Vitamin A it has, your hair will regrow.

A lack of protein

Too much Vitamin A can cause hair damage. But too little protein could also lead to hair loss. If your body isn't getting enough protein, you can ask for more. In order to ensure that the body receives enough protein, one way is to stop hair growth. It can happen within two to three weeks after your protein intake has been reduced.

Female hormones

Like the fact that hair loss can be caused by pregnancy, so too can hormonal changes in the bodies of females. This usually occurs when women first stop or try to use birth control. Women should be aware that birth control pills, like contraceptives can affect the hormonal balance. If your family history includes hair loss, then this disruption in the hormonal balance will be more noticeable and more likely. The hormonal changes that women experience during menopause can also affect their bodies. Also, this can lead to hair fall or telogen effluvium. Switching to contraceptives can help prevent this. However, it is better to talk with your doctor about the various contraceptives.

Trichotillomania

Experts have classified this behavior as a mental action. It is unclear whether this should be classified under obsessive-compulsive disorder or as a routine. However, one thing is certain: it can cause hair fall. Trichotillomania refers to the behavioral disorder that causes individuals with the condition to have an insatiable need for pulling or plucking their hair. It doesn't matter if the hair is on their head or arms or legs. Their main goal is to be able and able to alleviate their desire to pluck hairs. This can eventually cause a small cut or a wound that can be made into scarring. This would stop hair growth and would lead to common hair loss. It is important that the person suffering from this condition stops as soon as possible. Over time, hair regrowth might be possible. But, if the condition continues for a long period, permanent hair loss can occur.

Anemia

Research shows that anemia is a common condition which can lead to hair fall. Anemia is caused by the insufficient iron levels. This condition is very common for women aged 20 to 50. A doctor can do blood tests to confirm if you have anemia. If it is positive, then a change in your diet or supplement intake could reverse the damage. This is one reason hair loss is easy to treat.

Hypothyroidism

The thyroid gland is a tiny organ located just below the voicebox at the front. This tiny gland produces hormones that regulate our metabolism. It is vital to the body's metabolism as it regulates our growth and development. It can lead to hair loss, and possible hypothyroidism if the thyroid does not produce enough hormones. Hypothyroidism can also be called underactive thyroid. This could be due to autoimmune deficiencies, birth defects or surgery which may include the removal of the thyroid. Science has improved our future. Synthetic thyroid medication is now possible, which can restore thyroid hormone levels to normal.

Vitamin B Deficiency

Like Vitamin A, hair loss can also occur if our bodies lack Vitamin B. Although it is not common, hair loss can occur in very rare instances. The good news is that this can be fixed. You can solve your problems with Vitamin A and anemia by simply taking Vitamin A supplements and eating a nutritious diet. Vitamin B can be found on non-citrus fruits and vegetables as well as meat, fish, and meat.

Autoimmune Diseases

Poor immune system can lead to hair loss. This condition is known as alopecia arrea. This happens when our bodies become confused. The immune system perceives hair as something different or alien, and attacks it. Another type of this disease is arthritis or diabetes, which occurs when healthy body tissues are attacked. If this happens to our hair follicles, it can cause permanent hair loss as well as telogen efflium, which is a temporary disruption of hair's growth. You can alter this by taking some medications.

Infections

There are many causes of hair loss. Ringworms are the leading cause of hair loss. Many people mistakenly believe that ringworms actually are worms. This is false. Do not be misled by the name. Ringworm infection actually results from fungus. This condition is scientifically called Tinea capitis. This is due mold-like fungal species called dermophytes. These fungi have a favorite habitat in warm and moist areas. This can also happen to hair if you don't maintain good hygiene. This is more common with children, but can also occur to adults.

Chemotherapy

This is the first treatment that cancer patients should consider. Cancer cells can be dangerous cells that multiply and grow faster than normal cells. These cancer cells are stopped from growing rapidly by chemotherapy, which is why chemotherapy can be so effective in treating them. The bad news: cancer cells do not grow quickly in the body. The hair follicles also have a group of cells that are quick to grow. Exposure to radiation, such as chemotherapy, can cause hair loss and cancer cell destruction. When you stop being exposed to radiation from chemotherapy, your hair will regrow.

Dramatic Weight Loss

Although you may want to lose lots of weight, it is not healthy to do so by starving yourself or overtraining your body. There is no shortcut to getting to your fitness goals. It takes time and effort to get physically and mentally healthy. You can't gain the vitamins or minerals your body needs to function properly when you are starving. This can also lead to physical trauma if your body is exhausted too much. Both of these could lead to hair loss. Eating disorders such as anorexia or bipolar disorder can cause hair loss and weight loss.

Polycystic Ovary Syndrome

This only affects women, obviously. POS is a condition that causes an imbalance of the male and feminine sexhormones. Studies have shown that excess androgen can lead to infertility. When male hormones become too strong, women can have hair growth on their bodies and faces.

Medications

While certain medications can fix the problems that are causing your hair loss, some others may cause you to lose your hair. Blood thinners and antidepressants are common side effects of drugs that cause hair to thin. You might also experience hair loss from methotrexate (used to treat rheumatic diseases and skin disorders), lithium, and other antidepressants like ibuprofen. Your doctor should be consulted about your medications. If you suspect that your medication is causing your hair to thin, then talk to your doctor about lowering the dosage or switching to another medication.

The styling process

Thinning hair isn't just caused by braids or ponytails. When you want to look your very best, it is important to choose the right hairstyle for you. This can lead to lots of trial and errors, with many hair cosmetics, such as wax, gel and hairspray. This can cause scalp irritation, which could lead to a receding of the hairline. Our hair can be damaged by technologies such as hot-oiling, rebonding, and perming. Sometimes, hair can become damaged when it is exposed to heat or chemicals. This can affect the hair from the roots down. The roots may be damaged and your hair may not grow back.

Aging

Aging will always be a part of our lives. We will all age regardless of our wishes. As we get older, so does our bodies. This includes our hair follicles. The process of hair regeneration will change. Degeneration of hair becomes more apparent when women are 40- to 50 years old. Experts do not know why this is happening. This is why people choose to cover their thin hair with wigs, scarves, or other styles.

Anabolic Steroids

American Academy of Dermatology claims that hair loss can be caused by anabolic steroids. This is especially alarming for athletes who tend to abuse anabolic steroids in order to gain strength and muscle. Anabolic steroids are the same as polycystic or ovarian disease. This is the best way to get rid of the drug.

Chapter 2: The Right Ways To Cleanse And Condition Hair

You should provide the right conditions to allow your hair to grow quickly. It means that you feed your body the right nutrients, so your hair will grow naturally without any disruption.

For fast hair growth, you need to have healthy habits and change your styling and hair care products.

Use shampoos and conditioners that don't contain harmful chemicals

The problem with many drugstore shampoos is that they can actually damage your hair. These shampoos, conditioners contain ingredients that will prolong the shelf life of your hair or kill dandruff causing bacteria. They can also cause hair to fall out if they are too harsh on your scalp.

You should avoid two chemical surfactants in shampoos and conditioners: sodium laureth, also known as SLS, and SLES. They produce foam or lather that can easily be spread on the hair. These are extremely toxic and were reported by Environmental Working Group as causing skin irritation, organ poisoning, and cancer.

Other harmful ingredients found in shampoos include propylene glycol, isopropyl alcohol, and propylene glycol. They are added to shampoos to help with oily hair. It is so strong it will strip the hair's natural oils, proteins and prevent it from becoming brittle. Hair will eventually fall out or become thinner if they are used constantly.

You should also be on the lookout for another compound in shampoos. It is called Diethanomaline. Sometimes it is listed under the list ingredients as Cocamide DEA. It makes hair products creamy and is used in them. This product can cause cancer if it is used with other cosmetic products. According to the International Agency for Research on Cancer, the DEA reacts against the nitrites and can turn into nitrosamines.

Make sure to do extensive research online about shampoos, conditioners, and other products that are free of harmful chemicals. Check out reviews about these brands before you buy samples to try. A mild shampoo or conditioner is all that you need to gently remove dirt and oil from your hair while still maintaining the natural oils which keep it healthy and strong.

Always condition your hair after shampooing

Shampoo is primarily used to wash away oil and dirt buildup in your hair. This will protect your scalp from being irritated and causing dandruff. Your hair will also feel silky and clean, instead of feeling greasy. Shampoos are intended to remove oil so it is natural for shampoos also to remove natural oils which keep hair healthy. Here is where conditioner comes in.

A conditioner is basically a hair oil that restores the natural protective oils. Now, the next time you shampoo your locks, notice how it feels dry and rough. As a result, your hair will feel silky smoother after you have condition it. The conditioner should not be skipped as it can take some time for your hair to produce the oils needed to moisturize again.

It is important to find a conditioner that goes well with your shampoo. Manufacturers create special formulas that work together with a particular brand of shampoo. To help your hair grow faster, you would want to maximize the features of each product.

Learn How to Wash Your Hair Right

There is actually a proper way to wash hair. This method can prevent hair fall from breakage and dandruff. The correct way to shampoo your hair includes keeping your scalp clean. You should use the right shampoo, conditioner and styling products to keep your hair moisturized and clean.

Wash your hair and scalp by thoroughly wetting it. Point the shower nozzle at your head to ensure that your hair is thoroughly soaked.

Next, you need to apply shampoo to your hair. A cost-effective method to distribute shampoo on your hair and scalp is to fill a small plastic bottle measuring approximately 2 1/2 inches long and 1 1/2 inches wide with water. Next, squeeze the shampoo you desire into the bottle. You can then shake the bottle vigorously to distribute the shampoo evenly over your scalp. You should not apply shampoo to just one area of your scalp.

Apply shampoo to your scalp and massage it with the pads your fingers. Do not poke your scalp with your nails as this can cause irritation and infection. You can massage gently in circular motions starting at the top and working your way up to the ears and down to the nape. It is important to remove any deep-seated oil and dirt on the scalp. You should let the shampoo sit in your hair about one minute before you rinse.

A little conditioner can be applied to your hair before shampooing. Place a small amount on the palm of one's hand, then rub your hands together. Use your fingertips to apply conditioner to the hair.

You can then wash your face and continue with your normal routine. Next, rinse thoroughly the conditioner and shampoo.

After shampooing and washing your hair, you are ready to condition it with conditioner. You only need to condition your tips, which is the lower half, and not your entire hair. Because your scalp produces natural oils within hours of leaving the bathroom. This oil is distributed throughout your hair, not just the ends. Because of this, conditioning your hair from the root to the tip is a terrible idea. It will leave you with very greasy roots.

You can apply conditioner by placing a small amount in your palm. Then, rub your hands together. Use your fingertips to rub the product onto your hair. To distribute the product evenly, you can rub the hair tips between your fingers. Allow the product to sit in your hair for three-five minutes or until it dries completely, depending on how long the manufacturer recommends. After waiting, you can wash your rest of the body. For long hair, you can use a shower cap to protect your hair from the conditioner spreading around your neck and back.

Rinse your locks thoroughly. You can rinse your hair by bending down, then soaking it. This will keep the product from running down your neck as you wash it. Use of hair products can lead to acne.

Your hair should be rinsed well until it runs clear. After that, dry your head using a hair towel. Make sure to not wrap it too tightly. If you do not feel comfortable with a hair towel, you can wrap a towel around your shoulders to capture any water that has dripped from your freshly washed locks.

Deep-condition your hair every other week

You can keep your hair healthy and strong by deep conditioning it or applying a hair mask. A deep conditioner can strengthen your hair and prevent damage. Deep conditioners cannot reverse the damage. Hair is composed of dead cells. They are incapable of repairing and restoring themselves to their former state. A deep conditioner can prevent further damage.

There are many deep conditioning products. Again, make sure to choose products that are free from the harmful chemicals we mentioned earlier. You can make your very own hair masks by using natural ingredients. Check out chapter 6 to see some of the recipes you can make.

Chapter 3: Natural Treatments For 5 Most Common Hair Problems

Hair Loss

Natural hair loss treatments are best because they use natural ingredients. Natural hair loss treatments are different from any artificial treatments on the market today. They do not have known harmful side effects.

Researchers are currently studying different types and herbs to help prevent hair loss. Researchers have discovered that many herbs, including plants, can be used to stop hair loss or even grow hair back.

Properly nurturing your hair is key to keeping it healthy. Your scalp needs to have good blood flow.

It is important to remember that hair loss can be caused by many other factors. It could also be caused by hormonal imbalances, psychological stress, thyroid issues, hormonal imbalances, immune system disorders, medication, and other factors.

To treat hair loss, nutrition and the correct herbs are key. They can provide nourishment to the hair's follicles, which can then be revived and start growing hair again. There are many herbs which can be used to prevent and treat hair loss. Sesame oil and green tea are all good options.

There are herbs you can eat or drink and herbs you can use outside. Aloe vera is a good option to rinse your hair. Aloe vera will not only keep your hair healthy but will stimulate the hair's follicles.

Gray Hair

These simple steps will help you prevent your hair from going gray. You need to quit smoking. Cigarette smoking is one the most harmful things for our health. Healthy eating habits are essential to maintain a healthy lifestyle. You should eat the right amounts of meat, dairy, eggs, fish, and nuts. This will ensure that your body is nourished with healthy elements and vitamins. Oil masks, or any other homemade oil, can be used a minimum of once per week.

Another option is to color your hair with natural products. It is possible to color your hair with boiled tea leaves. While you might not see the final result immediately, this is the natural method.

Thinning Hair

Hot oil massages are one way to thin your hair. A hot mixture of two teaspoons oil and two tablespoons coconut oil can be used to massage the scalp for 15 minutes. After you have done this, you can begin to dry your hair with a towel that has been soaked in hotwater. To get a better result, repeat the process two to three times.

Castor oil is another type of oil that you can use to naturally reduce your hair's thinness. To use castor oil for your hair, heat a cup and rub it all over your scalp. After that, you can comb it. Wrap your hair in a towel, then wash the oil with natural shampoo.

Olive oil and honey may also be used for hair treatment. Combine a cup oil and 1 cup honey liquid and mix well. Keep the mixture for a couple of days. Then, use it on your hair and scalp. You can comb your hair, but not touching the scalp. After that, you should cover it with a tight showercap. Allow it to rest for at most an hour and then rinse it thoroughly.

Regular shampooing is good for hair. However, be mindful of the shampoo options you use. Stronger hair products can damage hair, so it's better to use mild shampoos. You could dampen your hair once a week during the summer, and then keep it conditioned. You can use rosemary water instead of just water.

Also, natural protein treatments can be very beneficial. Mix one egg yolk with one tablespoon of olive oil and one teaspoon vinegar. Allow it to sit on your head 10 to 15 minutes. Rinse it well.

Another thing you need to consider if your hair is to stop thinning is nutrition. Because hair is 100% protein, good hair growth is dependent on protein consumption. Meat, eggs, green dhal, soy and meat are all great sources of protein. Hair needs vitamins to grow healthy.

Dandruff

There are two types of reasons that we get dandruffs. Dandruff is caused by emotional stress, poor hygiene or too much fat. Excessive hair sprays use, infrequently using shampoo, and dry indoor heating are the external causes. Here are 6 helpful natural dandruff remedies you can make and apply at home.

Coconut Oil and Camphor

Apply coconut oil, neem oil, and camphor to your scalp. This would make natural dandruff management easy.

Hazel with Lemon

Mix 100g of witch hazel with 1 tablespoon lemon juice. You can then use this mixture for washing your hair. You can repeat this process until your hair stops shedding its dandruff.

Olive oil and almond butter

Mix almond oil and olive oil. Use the mixture to massage your scalp. Let it sit on your scalp for at least 5 minutes. Wash your hair well.

Shampoo for pain relief

Combine two tablets of aspirins with mild shampoo. Let it sit for around 2 minutes on your scalp. You should wash the hair as soon as the aspirin residues disappear.

Glycerin and coconut oil

Mix 1 tablespoon of vinegar, 1 tablespoon of glycerin (or coconut oil) and 1 egg. Then, combine them all until the mixture is a smooth paste. Then apply the paste to your scalp. Rinse your hair using shampoo. Rinse your hair with shampoo every seven to ten days.

Tamarind & Sugarcane

Combine some molasses in water and dampen the tamarind. After about an hour, rub the mixture on your scalp. Then wash it with shampoo. Do this once every seven days.

Brittle hair

First, you must realize that there isn't a quick fix for brittle hair. To treat brittle, you must have a plan. Otherwise, you won't be able solve your problems. A better hair treatment will come to you if you have a consistent routine. It is important to wash your hair frequently. Even though you can shampoo your head once a month, shampoo should be used every day. To stimulate blood flow to your scalp, it is possible to turn your head while shampooing. You can dry your hair with the towel after you are done. You should not blow dry your hair so it doesn't get damaged.

You may not know, but combing your hair regularly can make your hair brittle. You can treat brittle hair by brushing and comb your hair at least twice daily. A second therapy is scalp massage. You can add rosemary oil or sage to help. You will notice an improvement in the blood flow to your scalp if you gently massage it. Take good care of your hair roots. You also need to look after the ends. Split ends must be trimmed regularly.

Homemade hair masks can be very helpful for brittle hair. A hair mask made from ripe avocado can be made by smashing it and adding two tablespoons honey to the egg. You can apply this mask to your hair 20 minutes a week. Your scalp can also be massaged with amla or Brahmi oil for approximately 15 minutes. Additionally, you can make a fenugreek mixture by adding lemon juice to curd. These treatments are excellent for giving life to dry, brittle hair.

Chapter 4: Exercise and food

Chapter 1 highlighted two causes for premature hair loss that can be caused by health problems that can both be treated and diagnosed. However, it can be much more difficult to correct a health problem that is already identified. A pound of prevention is better that a pound cure. That is true for any illness or health condition that could lead to premature hair loss.

The body's hormone levels can be affected in many ways. Some can be controlled easily while others can't be. Chapter 1 identified two hormone imbalances that can lead to premature hairloss. The hormone imbalances are either an excess of androgens, or a deficit of thyroid hormones. It is difficult to say if hair loss is due to an imbalance in one or both of these hormones without medical testing.

You can take the necessary steps to promote healthy hormone production.

Androgen Hormones

Androgens is a group hormones that has the most direct impact on premature hair fall. They are produced by the sexual organs: the testes for men and the eggs for women. Genetics and age are not controlled, so the body's ability create these hormones in its sex organs will depend on how old you are. The adrenal cortex is the third source the body can use for androgens. The adrenal cortex produces hormones that regulate body health and well-being. One such hormone is dihydrotestosterone. This has been associated with hair loss. The health of the thyroid may also be affected by some hormones made by the adrenal complex, which could lead to premature loss. Preventing and treating early hair loss can be made easier by maintaining the health of your adrenal complex.

Exercise

Your body reacts to exercise in many different ways. The type and extent of exercise will determine which responses are healthy. Higher levels of androgens have been linked to certain types of exercises, including high-intensity. It can be difficult for some to draw a link between high intensity exercise, and premature hair loss. This is especially true with certain fads which attract both men and ladies to high intensity workout programs. Given the possibility that certain exercise programs could cause hair loss prematurely, it is important that you decide which form of exercise is more important. There are many ways to exercise that don't require high intensity, including low-impact aerobics like jogging and aerobics.

Diet

Research has extensively examined the impact of diet on adrenal complex and orrogen levels. Increased levels of the minerals vitamin D and zinc may be due to high levels of testosterone (an androgen). An unhealthy (lackingly consumed) amount of sugars or unhealthy (excessive), fat intake can lead to lower levels of insulin. Even excessive protein intake can lead to elevated androgens. Natural, balanced eating is the key to adrenal health. Do not consume supplements or excesses that can increase testosterone levels. It is better to eat balanced, nutritious meals that keep you satisfied between meals than meals that leave your stomach feeling bloated, hungry, or make you crave for more.

The Thyroid

Thyroid hormones don't have a direct correlation to hair growth. However, it is not necessary for them to do so. These hormones can be found in the thyroid gland. This gland is controlled by hormones made by the brain. The thyroid needs iodine. This element is part of a halogen family (the periodic table of elements) and it is present in both hormones made in the gland. Hypothyroidism can occur if there is insufficient intake of iodine. This refers to a lack or excess of thyroid hormones. Although it isn't clear exactly how lack of thyroid hormone can lead to hair loss or other symptoms, many studies have demonstrated that there is a clear connection. Hypothyroidism is not only linked to hair fall, but it can also lead to developmental disorders such as speech and movement difficulties, mental retardation and stunted growth. Women with thyroid problems, especially pregnant women, are at higher risk for stillbirth and miscarriage. In excess of iodine, hypothyroidism or a deficiency can result in hypothyroidism. Diet is the best way for the body to obtain its iodine supply naturally.

A doctor can confirm that there is a thyroid problem. Once a diagnosis has been made, you may need to take medication or dietary modifications. Regulating your intake of Iodine is key. Too much can lead hypothyroidism which can cause hair loss. Too little can also lead to hyperthyroidism that can cause thin, unhealthy hair. Thyroid problems may also manifest as hair loss and other symptoms.

These are some of the symptoms

list list-id="3" level="0" list-type="unordered">

Fatigue, weakness and hand shaking are all possible.

Nervousness and anxiety can lead to mood swings.

Rapid heartbeat, irregular or rapid

Dry skin

Difficulty Sleeping

Unexplained weight gain or frequent bowel movements

These symptoms could indicate that it's time to see a doctor about your thyroid health, and to reevaluate your diet.

Foods that are good for you

Adrenal health is dependent on a balanced diet. High quality fats and proteins from organic meats and fish are good for moderate consumption. Healthy magnesium levels will be maintained through seafood such as salmon and halibut, which are essential for a healthy adrenal cortex. As needed, you can include starches in your diet to boost energy recovery after exercising. But this should only be done in moderation. Organic fruits, vegetables and other foods will have lower harmful chemical contents. It is beneficial to eat fruits high in vitamin C such as citrus and cruciferous, or leafy green veggies. Vitamin B5 must be maintained in a balanced amount, as too many can cause overactive adrenal complexes.

Many of the foods that are good in the adrenal complex are also good on the thyroid. Seaweed, shellfish, kelp, and saltwater fish are all good sources of iodine. Good-old-fashioned iodized sea salt is also a good option. But it is important to use in moderation as excessive salt intake can raise blood pressure, which can be detrimental to adrenal health. You can get iodine from green vegetables, such as asparagus, Swiss chard, and spinach. Eggs and garlic also make good secondary sources. The best sources of zinc are beef, lamb, turkey, Brazil nuts, and sunflower seeds. These are all important for thyroid health. You should be cautious when using zinc. It can be linked to high levels of androgen.

It can be difficult to know which foods are good for your adrenal complex and which are bad for your thyroid. Oysters and other foods rich in zinc and/or iodine are not good for the adrenals complex. But there are plenty of sources of iodine. High intakes of vitamin D such as milk can cause damage to the adrenal complex. However milk is beneficial for the thyroid. While high levels of vitamin D can support thyroid health, excessive vitamin A can lead some types of hair loss.

Personal Review

A relative introduced me to this product when he purchased a package from a European country. I was told it was fantastic and that he was already experiencing signs of growth on his scalp. My cousin, who has suffered from genetic hairloss since an early age, has always had little or no hair. It was great to see him pleased with the results. However, if your hair is already completely bald it is not worth trying to stimulate regrowth. Use topical treatments to restore your full hair.

I did my research and ordered a container online. Even though the liquid felt refreshing and energizing on the scalp, one whole bottle was far too much. The liquid ran down my entire face. I also didn't notice any signs that my hair was growing back or strengthening. The cool sensation it gave me on my scalp made me decide not to spend anymore time or money on the product.

Chapter 5: What Causes My Hair Loss?

Jay London.

Before you can even start treating hair loss, you need to identify the root cause. There are many kinds of baldness.

Look for signs of hair loss.

Is your hair falling out in areas like the crown, temples or back, with only a small amount of hair visible on your sides and top? The common androgenic alopecia could be the cause, especially if it's a male.

Are there no bald spots with smooth edges? Are there no signs that scarring is occurring? This might be alopecia.

Is itching, burning or pain present in areas of hair loss? Is the scalp irritated or prone to bruising? Scarring alopecia is possible. Early treatment will minimize the damage.

Once you have established the type of hair loss you are experiencing you can check for other symptoms.

Are you suffering from severe emotional stress, or are you depressed? Did you have a recent operation or pregnancy, if so, what was it? Are you currently being prescribed heavy to moderate medications for a medical condition that is affecting your health? Telogen effluvium might be an issue.

Joint pains. Weakness in the chest, pain in the joints, pain in the mouth, headaches. These are the most common symptoms of lupus. Seek out a rheumatologist for help. Have your joints evaluated for signs of inflammation. A blood test can detect high levels anti-nuclear proteins in the blood.

Do you feel generally weak? Is your skin feeling a little paler than it usually is? Is your skin feeling cold in the hands and feet

Do you feel short of breath when you do any type of physical activity? These are indicators of iron deficiency. For confirmation of iron deficiency anemia, you will need to have a hematocrit (blood test that measures how many red cells your blood contains) performed.

Excessive acne, irregular periods and ovarian cysts may be signs of abnormal facial hair. You may have polycystic or ovarian syndrome. Check with your doctor to see if you have elevated testosterone levels.

Are you easily tired? Do you seem to be gaining weight too quickly even though your lifestyle and diet have not changed? Are you having trouble with concentration? Hypothyroidism may be a cause. Talk to your doctor about getting a blood test done to measure the amount thyroid stimulating hormone (TSH). If you have too much of this hormone, it could indicate hyperthyroidism.

Chapter 6: Healthy Diet

Here are some suggestions for healthy foods that will help you prevent hair loss.

Protein High. High in Protein. It is important to also consider where your protein comes from. Consider eating fish, beans and eggs as your source of protein, rather than pork and other high-fat foods. Avoiding hair loss is your goal. Steaks and other fatty foods which increase testosterone levels will not work. You should choose leaner meats, such as fish and chicken. Also, choose low-fat dairy products and, naturally, vegetables and soymilk. Soy milk and tofu are particularly high in protein, but lower in fat. These foods are great for preventing and treating hair loss.

Prunes. Prunes are rich in iron. This is a huge source for those suffering from hair loss and discoloration, hair dryness, hair fall, or hair dryness. Proper iron intake will immediately improve the hair's health. Other than prunes, green vegetables can also provide iron. This makes it more fun as there are many options for green and leafy vegetables. Because it has many benefits for the body, eating vegetables and fruits is one the best ways to fight hair loss. It is a great preventive method because it is good for the body and is less expensive than other hair loss treatments.

Carrots. A high intake of Vitamin A-rich vegetables like carrots will help to prevent hair fall. Healthy hair starts with healthy scalp. Healthy hair and scalp can prevent harmful bacteria from settling on the scalp and leading to hair loss. Healthy hair is not only possible with carrots. It is crucial to include carrots in a balanced and healthy diet that includes vegetables, fruits and whole grains as well as low-fat proteins, legumes and dairy.

Bean sprouts. In order to prevent hair loss, you should eat foods that contain silica. The body uses silica for the absorption of vitamins and minerals. It is important to remember that silica is needed for the body to absorb minerals and vitamins. Silica is found in potatoes, bean sprouts and cucumber skin. People often neglect many essential elements of their diets and can become confused. Even though they eat healthy food, it is not always enough to get the desired results. Silica is the key to this confusion.

Shrimps. If you are looking for alternative meats, there are plenty of options. One option is to eat shrimps. This is especially important to people who need to build muscles, and want to consume a lot of protein. Shrimps and other seafood is rich in Vitamin B12 as well zinc and iron. This helps to prevent hair loss and keeps hair healthy. In addition to this, the shrimps are great for your taste buds. It is possible to create many different recipes with shrimps or seafood. This makes healthy eating an enjoyable culinary experience.

Walnuts. Walnuts are known to be hair-friendly because of their high omega 6 fatty acid content. This is in addition to the high levels of Vitamins B1,B6 & B9, zinc, and iron. Walnuts are also high in protein making them a great source of healthy hair. However, balance is still important. Exercising walnuts in excess can have a negative effect. Some people may have a problem with selenium absorption from walnuts. Hair loss can be caused by too much selenium. It is important to use walnuts in moderation to ensure the highest nutritional value.

Oats. Oats have fiber. In order to have healthy levels of hair-friendly ingredients, it is important to include oats in your breakfast and snacks several times per week. It is incredible that the majority of ways to prevent hair-loss can be done through diet. Then, once you have successfully overcome hair loss through these methods, it becomes easier to continue with other areas of your body.

You can eat right and be healthy.

Chapter 7: Types and Common Symptoms of Hair Loss

There are several types of hair loss, each with different effects. Different treatment options are often required. Here are some:

Alopecia Areata - This is a form of hair loss that is primarily hereditary. But it is not contagious. It is possible to lose hair as hairless patches on your body. Spot baldness is sometimes called this. Hair loss may spread to your entire head in rare instances. This is the most common type in women.

Alopecia Totalis - This refers to a total loss of hair. This is often seen quickly and can sometimes be a progression of Alopecia Areata. While there is no definitive evidence to prove the cause of it, it has been determined that it is an autoimmune disorder.

Alopecia Universalis: This is the most severe type of hair-loss. All hair (including eyebrows) on your body, is rapidly lost. It is the most severe form alopecia areata. Alopecia universalis can affect approximately 1:00000 people in North America as well as Western Europe. This condition may be related to autoimmune disease.

Alopecia Barbae means that you lose your facial hair. Although most common in men it can also occur in women.

Alopecia Mucinosa (also known as follicular Mucinosis): It is inflammation-like in nature. It affects both hair follicle and the sebaceous cells (the pilosebaceous un). It usually causes no scarring and scarring hair loss. This can indicate the progression of scarring. Under a microscope, mucin can be seen around hair follicles in most cases. Most commonly, this condition affects the hair, scalp, and neck. In some cases, other areas of the body may be affected. Because hair can grow back if not treated immediately, it is crucial to be treated as soon as possible.

Androgenetic hair loss is also known as male-pattern baldness. While this condition is common in men, it can also occur in women.

This condition causes your hair to thin down gradually. For men, the condition begins with a receding forehead hairline. This condition affects around 50% of men. Also, men with Japanese or Chinese ancestry are less likely to be affected by this condition. However, it has been shown that men who smoke are at an extremely high risk for being affected by this condition.

Adrogenetic Adlopecia: This is also known by female pattern baldness. It is most common among women during menopause. The hair starts to fall out at the top, but becomes coarser on the scalp. In this instance, hair regrowth is possible because hair follicles remain alive. Hair does not recede in male pattern baldness.

Traction Alopecia. This condition is caused by excessive tension or pulling of the shafts due to hairstyles. This type is quite common in women. It can become irreversible if the condition isn't treated in time.

Anagen Effluvium (or anagen effluvium): This condition is often caused by the use of radiotherapy and chemotherapy as cancer treatment. It can be patchy or complete. It can grow back easily.

Telogen Effluvium (or excessive hair loss): This condition is more severe than the average. This condition is typically temporary and can be caused by stressful physiological and emotional events. These events include pregnancy, child births, severe emotional disorders, major surgery, and drug use.

Involutional Alopecia, a condition where your hair becomes thinner as you age. As hair that is not cut becomes very short, more hair cells move to the resting stage.

Many people believe they are experiencing hair loss when their hair strands start to fall off. It is possible for your hair to start thinning before it starts falling. If you're experiencing hair problems, you can seek out help during this phase and make the necessary adjustments.

We will discuss common symptoms that can cause hair loss to help you determine whether it is an issue.

3.1. Symptoms

Hair loss can happen in many different ways. This greatly depends on what the cause is. The sudden or gradual appearance of hair loss can be temporary. It could affect just your scalp, but it can also affect your entire body. You can lose your hair permanently or temporarily depending on the causes and how you treat them. Here are some signs and symptoms you might notice if your hair is falling out.

The gradual thinning of your hair on top of the head

This is the most common sign that hair loss affects men and women. Men often notice hair loss starting at their foreheads in a line pattern similar to an M.

Flaky or circular bald spots

Also, you may experience bald patches mostly the size of a coin. It is usually only on the scalp. Other times, this might be felt on the eyebrows or beard. If your hair is shaved, you may feel some itchiness or pain.

Full body hair loss

This condition may also be caused by medical treatment. Chemotherapy, which is the most popular cause of full-body hair loss, is also a leading one.

Hair thinning: In some cases, your hair might become too fragile to grow. This can cause it to break soon after it has grown out of the scalp. This will cause hair loss.

Now that you know what causes hair loss and how to recognize them, let's tackle hair loss permanently.

Chapter 8: How can you prevent hair loss

These are some of the most common steps you can take to prevent hair falling.

Avoid using your hair dryer often - it will cause your hair to dry out and can lead to hair fall.

Avoid hair straighteners or curlers. They are extremely hot and can lead to hair loss.

Avoid hair products that contain harmful chemicals. In some cases, they can cause hair loss.

If you're going to use a hair straightener to style your hair occasionally, be careful not to touch the scalp. If the scalp is burnt, the hair follicles may also be damaged. This will eventually lead hair loss.

You should only use the highest quality dyes on your hair. The dyes used in hair color can damage hair and cause hair loss.

Keep your hair loosely pulled. This will result in hair falling out and tension. Avoid hot rollers. These can keep hair strands in tension, which can lead to them breaking and falling down.

Natural ingredients are best for your hair. Today's shampoos are loaded with chemicals that can cause hair to fall if left unattended.

Even though it might seem tempting to brush your hair while it still is wet, you should not do so. Dry hair can be easily broken and you could lose a lot of hair.

Do not dry your hair with a towel. Too aggressive towel drying can result in hair being lost.

Consume good food to promote hair growth and stop hair loss. Fresh fruits and vegetables are a great choice, especially if they're rich in iron and zinc.

Hydrate well to maintain a healthy scalp.

Chapter 9: Different types of hair shampoos you can make at home

Everyone has different hair. Some have oily hair while others have normal hair. And some have dry hair. Hair products, coloring, curling and coloring can all damage hair.

Hair is made up two parts. The cuticle is at the outer end and the shaft is at the inner. The cuticle consists of layers that overlap, much like fish scales. These scales should be flat so that hair feels smooth and silky. If the scales open, hair feels dry and rough. This can happen for many reasons, including diet, stress, and health conditions. But shampoos also contain high levels of chemicals.

Here are nine hair shampoos worth considering.

Natural Shampoo Bar Soap

A century ago, all you needed to clean your hair and skin was a bar soap. It is possible to make your own natural shampoo soap by using castile soap. However, this may be too drying for your hair. Depending on your hair type (dry, normal, or oily), you can make your own shampoo soap with coconut oil and jojoba oil. This type of shampoo can be used on your hair as well. It also makes it easy to bring along liquid shampoo for travel.

Lemon Juice/Apple Cider Vinegar Wash

In the past, soap was too expensive so people used water and lemon to clean up the dirt and grime. The replacement for lemons was apple cider vinegar, which was cheaper than lemons. Apple cider vinegar has many wonderful properties. They can be used to smoothen hair, close the cuticles, treat itchy scalps, and improve blood circulation.

Simply add a tablespoon of apple cider vinegar to a cupful of water to make lemon juice or apple cider vinegar wash. Add another tablespoon to your hair if it is long. To make your own apple cider vinegar, cut an apple in half and then place the whole thing (skin, rings, core, and all) into a glass jar. Put the jar inside a dark cupboard, and let it sit for a few more weeks.

Baking Soda Wash with an Apple Cider Vinegar Rinse

All the chemicals found in haircare products and daily pollution can be removed by a baking soda shampoo and apple cider vinegar rinse. Use half a tablespoon of baking soda (also known to sodium bicarbonate), in one quart of water. After that, you can apply the paste to your hair. Rinse the hair with warm water.

Make a paste with 1 tablespoon of baking soda and some water. Then, gently massage the scalp. This will boost blood flow and also clean out the scalp's pores. A second jug with water and a tablespoon each of apple cider vinegar should be poured over your head. Followed by another jug with lukewarm.

Raw Egg Wash

Although eggs are an excellent source of protein, many people don't know that they can be beneficial to their hair. Just crack one egg and beat it until it's light and fluffy. Next, massage it into damp hair and down the scalp. It is then time to rinse it off with warm water. The apple cider vinegar rinse can be used to obtain the best results and get rid the "eggy smell".

Beer Wash

Beer, both nonalcoholic and alcoholic, should be used in the same way as apple cider vinegar. You will see a change in your hair's luminosity and body after using it. Hops, malt and other proteins have higher levels which can make your hair look healthy and strong again.

Be sure to have chilled the beer overnight before opening it. Just shampoo as usual, then add the flat beer to your hair. Massage it into your scalp. It will stay on your hair for several minutes. Rinse off with warm water.

Rice Water Wash

Rice water washes have been used for thousands upon thousands of years in Far East. Just cook the rice as usual, and then wash off the water with some water. Take the water out and put it in a clean container. Then add more water.

Coconut Milk Liquid Shampoo

You'll find your hair dry and brittle when you just wash your hair with liquid soap or a shampoo-bar. Castile soap should contain coconut milk. This will help prevent hair from becoming dry and brittle. Coconut milk allows oils to mix with water and makes hair soften than castile soap.

For coconut milk liquid soap you need to combine three tablespoons coconut soap and half a cup water. To add shine and moisturizing to your soap, you may also use essential oils. Two tablespoons coconut oil, or a tablespoon each of aloe verde gel.

You should be aware that this mixture can only last around a week. Therefore, make a batch and freeze it in smaller batches. Simply take out a couple of cubes one night before you are going to use it.

Milk and honey

The combination of honey and milk has been used for centuries to treat a wide range of beauty and health conditions. Make a shampoo that cleans, conditions, and moisturizes hair. Simply pour half a cup of milk in a container and then add two tablespoons honey. Shake well.

Dry Shampoo

You might find yourself unable to shampoo your hair due to a meeting late at night or a lack of hot water. Dry shampoos are available. Sprinkle the oatmeal or cornstarch on your scalp, then go through your hair. Let the oil draw in all the oils. It's best to comb it after it's been there for a while.

How to Thicken Natural Shampoo

Top Tip It's easy!

Important!

You need to be aware that hair must go through a transition period once you have stopped using store-bought shampoos. This could mean that your hair will feel oilier and may take between two and three weeks for it to return to normal pH.

Chapter 10: We Love our Hair

Hair loss can creep into our lives, no matter how hard we try. Today's hair loss has become more of a lifestyle problem than a condition that's governed by bad genes.

You might be surprised to know that we have more than a thousand hair strands. It is common for people to lose their hair on a daily base. On an average day we lose about 100 strands. This is not unusual. This is where the problem lies: those of use who can still grow at the least 100 strands each day go outside with a great mop of hair. Those who can't regain their lost hair will try any trick in order to hide the worrying problem of hair loss. It is not the solution to hair loss to wear caps all the time and to cleverly partition the hair to cover the spots that are bald. You can also manage baldness smarter.

Let's begin by listing the reasons.

Hair Loss: Causes

Androgenic, or male-caused hair loss, is the most common. This type is caused by hormonal imbalances.

This condition affects close 70 % of the male population.

Hair loss can happen in very unusual ways. The hairline gradually recedes from temples to the rear, but not entirely from sides or back. This is the "Hippocratic Wreath" which is a unique form of hair loss.

The maintenance of sexuality in men is dependent on the levels androgen hormones. This condition can lead to a general drop in androgen levels and androgen receptors. It also causes a decline in libido.

However, it is common to observe a paradox in which the same hormone that aids in the growth facial hair, suppresses hair growth at the temples.

Androgenic Areata: This is a type autoimmune disorder. It is often genetically passed down. Both men and women can be affected by this condition. The severity of the disorder will affect the amount of hair loss. One bald patch on one side of the head is the first sign. If the condition is severe, it can grow larger and lead to complete baldness.

This condition is estimated to affect only 0.1% to 0.20% of the world's population. In many cases, the condition appears in teenagers.

All autoimmune disorders are caused by an attack on one's own cells. The T lymphocytes in this case attack hair follicles. These cells are responsible under normal conditions for hair production.

It is also possible to lose hair in a diffused way, as opposed to starting with a single bald patch.

If there is a bald area, it can have a different shape than normal.

The underlying skin is generally healthy.

A unique aspect of this condition is the fact that hair can stop temporarily, then resume its growth. In most cases, the hair grows back. In rare cases, the hair may disappear entirely.

Stress is the biggest issue of our time and it must be dealt with. Because of society's norms, success and prosperity have been associated with physical attractiveness. Baldness, especially in men, is a delicate issue. Men who lose hair too early can feel depressed and isolated from society.

Hair loss is known to be caused by thyroid hormonal imbalances (hypo or hypo).

Hypothyroidism usually causes hair to fall at the frontal area. This is typically located in the third region of your eyebrow.

Children develop oval-shaped patches of hair near their temples. This is a very unusual pattern in hair loss. These bald patches may not contain any hair follicles. This condition is also known congenital triangle alopecia.

Nutrition: Good nutrition is the key to good health. Low iron metabolism, low levels of proteins, vitamins and micronutrients, as well as low iron metabolism have been associated with hair loss. Fast food with high amounts of animal fats, especially the liver is known to be high in vitamin A, which can lead to hypervitaminosis. It is no surprise that fast food has been getting a bad reputation.

Hair loss in men is also caused by infection. Teniacapitis, which is caused by fungal infections in which the fungus infects the hair shaft, can also cause severe hair fall in men. This form of baldness, known as tenia capitis, is easily communicable. Male baldness can also result from secondary syphilis, cellulitis, and dissection.

People who are taking regular medication for hypertension, blood pressure, diabetes, hormone corrective therapies, contraceptive pills, and diabetes can also be at risk of hair loss. Cancer patients undergoing chemotherapy are also at risk of hair fall.

Hair loss can also occur due to hair manipulations by individuals. Hair loss can also be caused by hair damage such as excessive blow dryer use or vigorous combing.

A psychological disorder where pulling one's hair becomes an obsession can cause hair loss. Trichotillomania, a psychological disorder, is the name for it.

Trauma from parturition or surgery can disrupt the cell cycle and cause it to become disturbed. This causes a sudden stoppage in their cycles and allows them to enter the resting period. This condition is also known by telogen effluvium. Patients who have undergone chemotherapy for cancer may also experience this condition. Normal hair follicles can become affected and eventually lead to hair loss.

Hair loss can also occur when radiotherapy is administered to the head in certain cancers.

Hair loss is also common in body builders that use steroidalhormones.

Exposure to sunlight can lead to severe hair loss. The phototoxic effect, which is the sun's damaging effect on hair follicles, is also known.

The majority of people experience hair loss as they get older. The resting phase, or telogen phase in the cell cycle, is where hair follicles begin to lose their hair. The hair doesn't grow anymore.

It is crucial to keep your scalp healthy. Cosmetics like sebum, and other enhancing cosmetics, can cause more damage than good to hair follicles. They are more likely to become blocked, and hair won't grow anymore. Clogging can also occur due to environmental toxins in water or air.

Chapter 11: Hair Fall and Loss

Alopecia is the scientific term for hair fall. However, there are several types, with different effects and symptoms. It may surprise you to know that hair fall can also affect children. There are many types of hair loss that can affect children as young as 10 years.

There are many possible causes and treatments for each type. This is why it is so important to get to know them all. Knowing which type of hair loss is affecting you will make it easier for you to choose the right treatment.

We have listed all types of hair-loss problems that both children and adult can experience.

Telogen Effluvium

This type of hair fall is temporary. It occurs when large numbers of your hair reach the end of their lives. You may experience hair shedding (or hair thinning) in specific areas of the scalp. This happens when your body suddenly changes.

Androgenic Alopecia

This type of hair fall is genetic. This condition can affect both women and men. It is known as "male baldness," and can be seen in both men and women. The condition is known as "male-pattern baldness" for women. This will be apparent by their 40s.

Most men will experience androgenic orlopecia, which manifests in a receding hairline starting at the crown and going down to the frontal area. Women's hair tends to thinning across the entire head, with the crown experiencing the greatest loss.

Trichotillomania

This type of hair loss occurs mostly in children. This happens when a patient suffers from a psychological disorder. Stress or anxiety can trigger the hair loss.

A habit formed from emotional stress. The symptoms are still present and can cause hair loss.

Involutional Alopecia

This type of hair loss occurs naturally. This happens due to the life cycles of the hair follicles. Although hair falls gradually, strands will tend to thin as they age. As we get older, the last phase in our hair cycle will see more hair follicles. Although new hair will emerge, they will be shorter and smaller.

Alopecia Universalis

When all of your hair falls out, this is called hair loss. This can happen to your eyebrows and eyelashes as well as your eyebrows and pubic hair. This is a sign of an illness and should be treated medically.

Alopecia Areata

This kind of hair fall can affect both adults as well as children. The appearance of bald spots can cause patches to appear and eventually lead to total baldness (alopecia completeis). 90% of people with this condition are able to get their hair back after a few more years.

HAIR FALL FALLACIES, FREAKOUT POINTS

We have already said that hair fall doesn't necessarily mean hair loss. We usually shed hair on an almost daily basis. There are times when you shed hair several times per day. This is not something to worry about. Next time someone tells to you that you shouldn't be losing hair, remind them that even hair goes through a life cycle. The next time they tell you otherwise, let them know it is natural. Don't panic at this point.

When you see signs of baldness out of the blue, it means that your hair is not dying too quickly or falling out. If any of these symptoms are present, it is time for a professional.

You should not attempt to treat the problem if you have reached old age, which is 60+. Although the reason for this is unknown, it is still dangerous to try any remedies.

For fashion, however, you have other options. To cover your bald spots, you could wear scarves and hats or even wigs. You don't have to do this if it is too bothersome.

You can have thick, healthy hair, even as you get older. This will be discussed in future chapters.

In the meantime you can examine your hair fall to determine whether it is an indication of panicking or just a natural process. It is best to examine your scalp, crown and frontal scalp. These are the most thinned areas on your head. A sign of hair loss is visible hair that cannot be seen clearly on your scalp. Find out if your hair type matches any of the descriptions.

Chapter 12: Foods and Drinks that Lead to Hair Loss

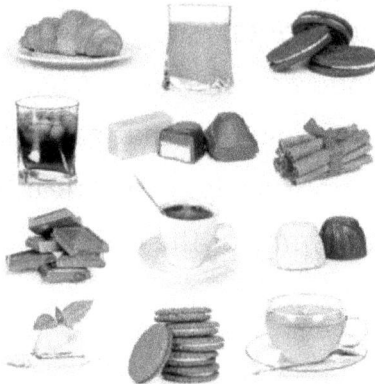

If you want to grow healthy and long hair, there are many foods you should avoid. You will lose vital minerals such as calcium, vitamin C, iron, omega-3 fatty acids, vitamin D, and vitamin B. These foods are best avoided.

1. Sugar

Sugary foods, such as sweets, should be avoided because it can hinder the absorption protein, an important building block in hair growth. Sugar is very acidic and can cause damage to B vitamins in the body. It also lowers concentrations of other minerals, which directly interferes with hair growth. Indirectly, hair loss is also caused by refined carbs like bleached bread and flour high in sugar and fiber. Refined carbs, such as bleached flour, can reduce the body's ability for stress management. This is one of the main factors that can lead to hair fall. Telogen Effluvium (a physiological stress disorder) is the name for stress-related hair fall. It results in hair shedding or thinning. Avoid sugary cereals or processed carbs. Instead, try honey or stevia as natural sugar substitutes.

2. Additives for food

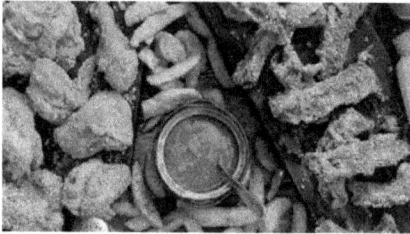

A number of synthetic ingredients, including caramel color, can cause hair loss and stunted development. This is mostly due to ammonia, which is processed by sulphite, or other caustic chemicals. Your hair can be affected by a few natural additives like carmine color extract which is made from dried bugs. Carmine dye may cause hair loss, and possibly allergic reactions that can seriously affect people.

3. Fried Foods

Foods containing high levels fats (e.g. fried foods) are also to be avoided. Consuming high amounts of saturated or monounsaturated fats can increase Dihydrotestosterone levels (or DHT), which can lead to hair loss. DHT levels are higher in men than women, and this is thought to lead to androgenic alopecia (male-pattern baldness). The US has 50 million males and 30 million females who experience hair loss as a result of androgenic and hormonal alopecia. Consuming hydrogenated oils reduces the essential fatty acids needed for hair growth.

4. Soft Drinks and Alcohol

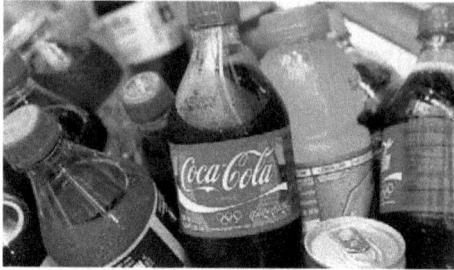

A low level of zinc and vitamin B and C in your hair is a major problem for long-lasting healthy hair. Insufficient minerals can cause weak hair, slow growth, and hair loss. Soft drinks like soda can contain high amounts sweeteners, food coloring, high fructose syrup, and processed Sugars. These additives can damage hair growth and cause it to become dry and brittle. Carbonated drinks can also be high in artificial sugars, which triggers insulin resistance. This condition is where the body cells cannot respond to hormonal insulin. Research suggests that baldness, which is an indicator of insulin resistance, can also signal high blood sugar levels. To reduce hair loss, hair thinning, and stunted growth, you should cut back on the consumption of soft or carbonated drinks.

5. Greasy Foods

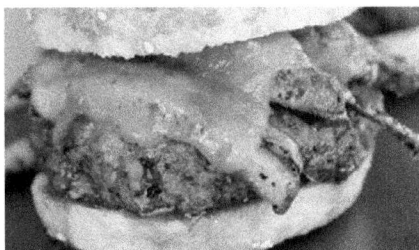

These foods can cause clogging in your arteries and greasy skin growth on your scalp. The buildup of greasy hair on your scalp can lead to slow blood circulation and clogging the pores and hair follicles. DHT hormone gets trapped in this way, which can lead to baldness. Even though shampooing your hair may help remove some grease, eating non-grease foods like natural fats or oils is the best option. You should avoid eating prepackaged food like fries, popcorn, or any other prepackaged food. The extra salts can cause hair loss and damage to your body. Excess sodium can lead to hair fall.

6. Processed dairy

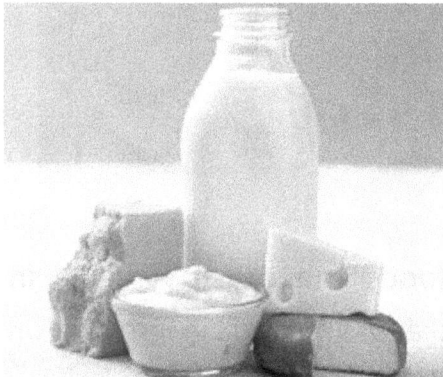

High fat, processed daily, can cause hair damage. Acidic digestion creates an acidic atmosphere in the body which can cause allergic reactions. Pasteurized dairy eliminates the natural enzyme found in milk. It is responsible for the digestion of milk. Without this enzyme, milk that is taken into the body does not benefit the cells. It's instead broken down by harmful bacteria, which causes the buildup of toxic substances in the blood. Processed dairy by-products can cause skin pores to clog, which can lead to epidermis plaque buildup and hair loss. Consume only unpasteurized, unsweetened dairy to reverse hair fall and encourage the growth of long, healthy natural hair.

Chapter 13: Simple Ways to Prevent Hair Fall & Reduce Its Impact

Proper Care:

To keep your hair healthy and prevent further damage, it is vital to properly care for it. It is better to wash your hair on an every other day basis than once per week. This will preserve some of the essential oils and help promote the hair shaft's strength. You should also avoid over-styling. Avoid over-styling with a blowdryer. Keep it at least six inches from your scalp. Do not style your hair with tight braids or pony tails. To lessen the tugging on your hair shaft, you can use a wide-toothed combing instead of a brush. Use heat-resistant styling products only. Avoid any chemical dyes or straightening agent that can cause hair loss. Make sure you properly condition your hair. You can even use an intense weekly conditioner.

Good Diet:

In order for hair to grow strong and healthy, it needs proper nourishment. Healthy hair requires a healthy diet rich in protein, fruits, and vegetables. A multi-vitamin supplement will provide you with any other nutrients that your body is lacking. You should eat a full meal when taking your vitamin to increase its absorption.

Reduce Stress:

Stress should be minimized in your life. This is something that can be difficult, but it is important. Your body will be in balance if you take a relaxing bath at the beginning of each day or get weekly massages.

Refusing to Pay the Loss

While the solutions that we have presented will work, it may take time. While you wait for hair to grow, there may be some ways to conceal hair loss. Let's examine the two most common.

Wigs:

For centuries, the number one way to cover hair loss has been with wigs. Wigs today can be virtually undetectable. It is best to get a quality human-hair wig. It is crucial to make sure that the wig you purchase is properly fitted and of good quality. Chap wigs might not allow airflow through hairs and caps. This could reduce the oxygen in your hair and make your hair loss worse. Badly fitted wigs can increase pressure on the hair and lead to more hair loss. You should ensure you buy a quality product and that it is professionally fitted.

Hair Building Fibers:

Hair Building fibers are one of the most popular cosmetic treatments for hair loss for women. Hair building fibers work best for those with diffuse hair loss. Hair building fibers are available in many cosmetic stores and online. These fibers are typically made of colored protein keratin to match your hair color. Static electricity within the fibers attaches to your existing thin hair and makes it look thicker. They are almost always invisible. They are also resistant to wind and rain, but can be easily washed out with regular shampooing. They are quick fixes that can instantly make your hair look great with very little effort.

Hair Transplants

Before you go to the surgeon, try natural methods or medications. If you're still not satisfied with the results, then hair transplants may be an option. A hair transplant is often a great option for women because they can often cover any scalp scarring caused by it. Grafts are a permanent solution for hair loss. In the next sections, we'll discuss the 2 main types hair transplant surgeries.

Follicular unit Transplantation (FUT):

FUT is a more traditional method for hair transplantation. FUT uses a horizontal strip of scalp that is cut from the lower portion of the skull. The strip can then be dissected into individual transplants.

FUT's Pros

- You can cover more areas of hair loss in a shorter amount of time

- The grafts can be more successful because they stay attached to your scalp for longer.

Lower Cost

.

Follicular unit extraction (FUE):

FUE is a modern technology that extracts individual hair units from the rear of the head with a specialized tool. FUT creates a scar, but this method doesn't leave a large one. This process takes longer but it's generally painless thanks to the use of numbing medicine. The process is much quicker because it does not involve a large wound.

FUE: The Pros

- No large, straight scar on the scalp's back

- Recovery is quicker

FUE extraction is most commonly used for women. Because women have smaller areas that are bald and prefer to avoid scarring, FUE is a popular choice. The procedure is gentle enough to be comfortable for women. But, before you make any decisions about your case, it's best to consult your doctor.

Laser Treatment to Grow Hair

If you find hair transplant surgery too painful, laser treatments could be an alternative. Lasers can help stimulate hair growth. Lasers are gaining popularity with cosmetic surgeons. You can use a low light laser to apply a comb or helmet on your head. There are even systems that can be used in your own home. Laser therapy is commonly used for hereditary male pattern baldness. Like any other treatment, success rates vary.

Hair lasers are able to stimulate hair growth in the following ways:

- Increasing the blood flow to your scalp

- Lower inflammation of the scalp

- Stimulating the cell metabolism

- Reducing effects of protein-blocking proteins

Chapter 14: Herbal hair loss treatments

Natural herbs are a rich source of medicinal herbs. Certain herbs show effective results against hair fall. Here are the details of some herbs, along with how to treat hair fall.

Ginkgo biloba

This herb belongs in the Ginkgoaceae group. Ginkgolides B, C and J, M are the most effective bioactive phytochemicals in this herb for treating hair loss. Ginkgo biloba combined with these bioactive phenolics improves microcirculation within the cerebral portion of the brain. This oxygen supply is sufficient to support hair growth.

Direction: Combine Ginkgo Biloba and coconut oils. Let the mixture boil for about a minute to extract the herb content. Turn off the heat. Then let the mixture cool. The mixture should be kept in an airtight, glass bottle. You can achieve a great result by massaging the mixture into your scalp at least twice a night. [3]

Phyllanthus embelica

This herb belongs to the Euphorbeaceae. It also contains phyto-ingredients including phyllemblin, and tannin. This herb is rich in Vitamin C as well as minerals such iron, calcium and even phosphorous. Hair loss is often caused by iron deficiency. Iron content in hemoglobin provides oxygen to different parts. Combination of bioactive phytochemicals and nutrients makes this herb ideal to treat hair fall. The iron content of this herb aids in oxygenating hair follicles. It also supports hair growth. Sometimes oral intake may not be sufficient to provide all the nutrients necessary for hair follicles. External application of this herbal remedy aids in hair growth.

Direction: The common name of this herb, Indian gooseberry, is the most common. You can dry enough gooseberries and then mix the coconut oil. Boil this mixture. Cool it completely. You can store it in a glass bottle. Once ready to use, mix equal amounts of mixture with lemon zest. For hair growth and prevention of hair loss, apply the shampoo all over your scalp. [3]

Allium cepa L

Liliaceae is the common name for onion, a common herbal ingredient. This herb is rich in phytochemicals. These include albumin (protein), alliin. Alliin, allylpropyldisulphide. Allicin. Diallyl sulphide. These phytochemicals support hair growth. You will also find various minerals in onion, such as zinc, magnesium, potassium, trace amounts of chromium and calcium. Zinc stimulates oil glands and helps to prevent the scalp from drying. This could help to prevent hair damage from dandruff. Iron aids in red blood cell production, and helps maintain blood circulation. These factors are important for hair growth.

Direction: Apply onion liquid to any patchy or bald areas. This will give you the best results. Experts recommend that you apply onion juice twice daily to the bald spot. If the area becomes reddish, massage it with honey. Then rinse off with cold, clean water. [3]

Lavandula angustifolia Miller, Rosmarinus officinalis

Lavender oil extracted form Lavandula angustifolia Miller is used in hair loss therapy. Rosemary oil extracted by Rosmarinus Officinalis is also used. These medicinal herbs both belong to the Labiatae famiy. Both of these medicinal herbs contain essential bioactive phytochemicals which can help support hair growth. The phytochemicals in rosemary oil include borneol 1, 8-cineole bornylcetate, cineols, lavendulyl.acetate and linalyl.acetate. Rosemary oil also contains 1-2% of volatile oil, and its chemical structure contains between 0.8 and 20% of esters.

These active phytochemicals can easily be absorbed by massage and inhalation. These oils stimulate the senses and promote circulation. Oils can also be inhaled, which allows them to penetrate into the skin. These oils can reach the receptors and change the pathophysiological circumstances that are associated with hair loss. A combination of these oils has been used on hair roots to stimulate hair growth. It can also be used for hair loss treatment. This is the reason why essential oils are not well understood.

Direction: Use a blend of these oils for a gentle massage on your scalp. This will support hair growth. The therapy should be maintained for at most 7 months in order to produce an effective result. [3]

Juglans regia L.

This herbal remedy, also known as Walnut, is a common name for it. Walnuts contain the perfect mix of fatty oils that promote hair growth. The fatty acid compositions of walnuts include 50.58-66.60% Linoleic Acid, 14.88-28.51% Oleic Acid, and 9.16-16.42% Linolenic Acid. As a trace, this herb contains other fatty oils in addition to these major fattys. Nuts also contain calcium, magnesium potassium, phosphorous, and sodium as chemical constituents. Micro-constituents also included in this herbal product are iron, zinc. copper. manganese. Potassium is found in the kernels and seeds of nuts.

Nuts are rich in essential minerals that increase hair growth. As iron is a carrier of oxygen and promotes circulation, it can also help supply oxygen to hair roots. Zinc stimulates oil glands. It also maintains an oil balance in hair's follicles. This prevents hair loss and scalp dryness. Tripeptide complex aids in hair regrowth and hair loss. The effectiveness of the Tripeptide Complex is high, and it can help to reduce hair loss due alopecia. The walnut's copper content improves the tissue level, and helps maintain the healthy balance of the mineral. Its concentration is between 1.7mg-3.5 mg.

Direction: Walnut oil, which is extracted from walnuts, can be found in supermarkets and markets. Place organic, unadulterated oil into a small bowl. Massage the oil on your hair roots. It will nourish your hair roots, and help you grow hair. [3]

Glycyrrhiza glabra Linn

This herb is a member the Leguminosae and contains several bioactive components, including glycyrrhizin. Research has shown that these phytochemicals from licorice have a hair-growth promoting effect.

Direction: Mix licorice pieces and saffron milk together to create a paste. Next, apply to the baldness in bed. Then wash your head. You will see an improvement in your results if you continue with this therapy. [3]

Ricinus communis

This herb is part of the Euphorbiaceae plant family. This herb's beans can be used to extract castor oil. It also contains Ricinoleic acids, which have the potential to increase Prostaglandin E2 synthesis in the scalp. Numerous supporting documents suggest that increased Prostaglandin E2 synthesis in the scalp can help increase hair growth. It also has the potential to treat baldness and alopecia.

Direction: Apply oil to scalp and massage lightly. This helps to increase hair growth. You can also apply this to any area where there is no hair. [9]

Chapter 15: Hair Combs and Brushes:
Types of Combs

The type and material you use to comb your hair depends on its length and structure.

The most common materials used in the production of combs and brush are:

Plastic. Plastic combs cost less, are easy to clean and are hygienic. They can be used on any length of hair. The plastic cracks can cause hair to tangle if you give it a gentle blow.

Metal. Metal combs work well for short haircuts as well as for splitting the hair into strands or untangling long curls.

They can cause injury to the scalp so they are not recommended when you are combing thin, colored or damaged hair. Each metal tooth must be covered with a ball containing silicone, rubber, and plastic. Hair dryers can damage hair, so it is best to avoid using a metalcomb. But, metal combs are practical, durable, long-lasting, easy to clean, and don't electrify your hair.

Natural bristles. Natural bristles are made from horse, pork and whalebones. The natural bristles of brushes and combs have many advantages. They don't react with cosmetics, remove static electricity, can be used to massage the scalp, add sebum to the hair and protect it from any damage. Natural bristles brushes and combs don't allow for a good hairstyle.

Wood. The most useful combs made from wood are those that are made. You can identify quality wooden combs easily by their smooth handles. They don't have a rubberized base, glue or lacquer smell, but instead they smell like the tree from where they were made. You should choose a comb from hardwood like sandalwood, oak, birch, and the juniper.

Wooden combs can add shine and silkiness to hair.

The fungus can grow on wood surfaces so you must clean it up regularly. They can also be quite fragile and cause allergic reactions.

Silicone. Silicone combs have the appearance of a mixture of plastic and rubber. They are easy-to-clean and highly hygienic. Silicone hair combs can be used with wet hair. They can be used without static electricity to untangle hair naturally. They can be used for a very long time. Silicone does not release any harmful substances when hair is dried using a hairdryer.

Carbon. Carbon is an artificial alloy and contains microfibers of graphite or rubber. Combs can be used for all hair types. Ceramic coating protects carbon combs. They do not require any special care and will retain their quality and neat appearance for a very long time. Carbon combs offer high strength and resistance to high temperatures, as well as antistatic properties.

Nylon. Nylon brushes offer a cost-effective alternative to bristles made from natural hair. They can be used for styling or straightening hair.

Nylon brushes have low prices and are very hygienic. They are long-lasting and can be used to extend hair or massage scalp. It is safe to use on the scalp and hair strands.

However, it isn't ideal for curling long hair.

Ebonite. Ebonite is a long-lasting material with black or brown colors. It is produced by the vulcanization and sintering of rubber. It is widely used in the manufacture of professional combs.

Ebonite is a great comb for coloring hair and perming.

Its drawbacks include the fact that it can soften after washing in hotwater and the possibility of color change if the ebonite is left out in direct sunshine.

Ceramics. Ceramics means the best comb, since it doesn't electrify.

Many modern models come with an ionization feature that simplifies and speeds up the process of hairstyling. The ceramic coating can be heated evenly while drying with a hairdryer. A ceramic comb is also available with tourmaline coating.

However, care is necessary because of its fragility.

Types of brushes and combs

Make sure to consider not only the material but also their structure and shape when choosing a comb or brush for your hair.

Massage brush. A massage brush consists of a base, and a full-handle made of plastic or wooden. The working surface of massage brushes is typically rectangular with rounded corners. The base contains a rubberized coating or textile that fixes the teeth. Massage combs may be made from natural bristles (or plastic), or metal. The length of the tooth is 0.4 or 0.8 inches (1 or 2. cm).

The advantages of message brush include improved blood supply to hair and follicles, increased sebum distribution along the length of the hair, and good care.

The downside to this is the gradual accumulation and buildup of dust and skin oils on the surface. Therefore, it is important that the massage brushes be regularly cleaned and disinfected.

Round Brush. A handle and a base are the basic components of the round brush. The base is made of either wood, metal or ceramic. The teeth can be made of nylon, nylon bristles, metal, plastic, and horse or pig teeth with balls at both ends. There are also round brushes that have mixed teeth. They contain both natural bristles, and plastic teeth.

Round brushes offer multifunctionality. They are able to add volume to hair near the roots while styling, curl and straighten hair, as well as stretch and curl hair ends.

They can be hard to keep clean.

Semi-round brush. It is a semi-round brush that has a convex shape base with 7-12 rows of tooth. The semi-round bases mean that the teeth are not as close together.

This brush is ideal for styling medium and short haircuts, such bobs or quads. A semi-round round brush can be used to curl fringes and massage scalp.

However, electrification is possible if the semi-round toothbrush's teeth are made out of plastic.

"Fishbone". The primary purpose for the skeleton toothbrush is to give the hair extra volume. It is also known as the "fishbone", or "skeleton" toothbrush because it resembles the fish skeleton. It has holes in the base, and teeth made of plastic or silicone. This type is used for hair drying.

The brush's base is designed to allow air to circulate through it, which makes drying hair dry faster.

Do not use the "skeleton" brush to dry and brittle your hair.

Flat comb. The flatcomb has a broad rectangular base where the teeth are located. It's the best comb to use for long hair.

Even thick hair can be combed with ease by a broad base and frequent, regular teeth. It's gentle on hairs and doesn't break them.

It's also difficult to clean and can electrify the locks.

Crest. Crests can either be made from wood, horns, or bones of animals, or from plastic, metal alloys.

They are convenient for using to cut and straighten ends of hair.

However, crests can be fragile if they are made from plastic. This makes them inconvenient when combing long hair or curling.

Brush. For long curls, the brush will be the best choice. This brush can be used for smoothing and finishing hairstyles. This type can be made with either artificial or natural teeth.

Tangle Teezer hairbrush. Tangle Teezer hairbrush has convex shape. It fits comfortably in the arm.

The brush offers many advantages, including the fact that it isn't harmful to hair; it's portable; you can use it for all types of hair, natural and long; it doesn't damage the hair structure and scalp; and it doesn't generate static electricity.

It can be used to treat dry hair as well as wet hair.

Be aware that there are many fakes.

Straighten hair using a hairbrush The long clip makes it easy for you to straighten hair. Manufacturers recommend it for use while drying hair with hair dryer.

This comb offers many benefits: it doesn't damage hair; is compact; locks securely and won't slip during straightening.

The disadvantages are: they can be fragile.

Specialized hair combs

* Infrared. The overall nutrition of the hair is optimized when using an infrared combing device. As a result, oily seborrhea, dandruff, and oily seborrhea disappear and the strands are stronger and more resilient. It is helpful in cases where hair loss has occurred. A doctor consultation is required before you use an infrared-comb.

* Ionic. Combs that use ionization to produce static electricity are intended to smoothen hair and give curls smoothness.

* Laser. This comb encourages hair growth, combats alopecia, reduces static electricity and improves blood flow. You should consult a doctor before using the laser comb.

* The ironing comb has the ability to straighten your teeth. It looks just like an ordinary brush but has teeth on the working surface. For hair protection, protect the hair from thermal damage.

* Hairdryer-comb (thermal brush). It looks like a normal round brush. It's not like the usual round brush. The ceramic base of comb-hairdryer has a hollow bottom. The thermal brush has a lower hair-drying effect than a hairdryer.

* With the effects of massage. The hairbrush-massager is safe for your hair. It activates dormant follicles of hair, fights with electrified, normalizes production of sebum and helps with headaches.

Choosing A Comb By Hair Type

* Long. A suitable flat comb and brush, with 12-15 rows. A large brush is used to twist the tips of the hair and increase the volume in the root. You should discard crests with too many teeth as it can be difficult to comb long hair.

* Medium. It is recommended to use a medium-diameter and semi-round brush.

* Short. * Use accessories with shorter teeth. For volume, you can use the "fishbone", or small-diameter toothbrush.

* Wavy. A natural brush with bristles will add style and charm to your hair. If you find the waves too stiff, you can use the comb straightener.

* Curly. This comb will fit well with long, rare teeth. It is best to get rid of the "fishbone" and use a crest that has frequent, short teeth.

* Kinky. You might like a crest or comb that has rare teeth.

* Straight. Any comb works.

* Soft, thin, fluffy. You can use a round brush to style and a regular brush for everyday usage.

* Thick, hard. Choose products that have flexible, rare teeth. Use a comb made of a hard but delicate material such as silicone, ebonite, or carbon. Do not use thick bristles or natural bristles on your brush.

* Rare. * Rare. For more visual volume, you can use the round, semi-round or fishbone brushes.

* Oily. For a decrease in sebum production, it is best to avoid over stimulation. Avoid using a massage brush. Instead, use natural bristles on combs. A wooden crest with frequent teeth can be used to manage oily hair.

* Dry, brittle. Get rid of the metal brush. Replace the metal comb by one with natural bristles and silicone teeth, like the Tangle Teezer Brush.

* Extension hair. You should use a medium-large brush for combing or a brush made of natural bristles.

How to Choose the Right Comb for Your Purpose

* Comb for hair style. A semi-round and round brushes, as well as a brush with a diameter suitable for hair styling, are all acceptable.

* For volume. Use a brush, a "fishbone", and a sponge.

* Reduce static electricity. The best versions are ionic or wooden.

* For gloss or polishing. For polishing there are separate devices such as Split Ender combs. You can also add gloss to your flat

brush by using a lot of natural bristles, or teeth.

* For soft combing. Use a Tangle Teezer and silicone brush.

* For hair straightening. The best ironing comb and thermal brush are effective. You can use a brush to avoid creating too much tension while combing.

* For bouffant. The crest should have long, thin and frequent teeth. The second variant of the bouffant comb has teeth with different lengths and is placed in 2-3 rows.

* To untangle. A flexible tooth brush is the best option. It can be a Tangle Teezer comb or a silicone one. You shouldn't attempt to solve tangles using a comb that has frequent teeth if they are quite complicated.

* For curls. You can twist curls with a heat or bristle brush.

* Don't dry your hair. If you have to comb right after shampooing your hair, you can use a Tangle Teezer (or a fishbone) comb.

Important Nuances

A key to success is selecting the right type of comb. Keep your comb clean and in good condition to ensure it will last a long time. Here are some useful tips for how to care your comb.

* You should never give the comb out to anyone. This is the same personal hygiene item you would use to brush your teeth.

* Get rid of hairs that are stuck between your teeth every day. For these purposes, you can use an older toothbrush. Brushing your teeth with a toothbrush will remove dirt from the bristles. After washing the comb, rinse and dry it.

* Wipe your hairbrush with mild soapy solution at least once every week.

* Avoid storing wooden products near heaters or high humidity locations.

* Wipe any grease or dust off the comb using hydrogen peroxide (mild-antiseptic) and other appropriate antibacterial products. After that, wash the comb well with plenty of water.

* Do not wash ebonite pieces in very hot waters. This will cause the material to soften and deform.

* If you see cracks or burrs in your teeth, replace the comb.

It is not easy to choose the right comb. It's possible to find the best comb if your research reveals the many styles and materials available.

Natural materials are best for brushes and combs. I highly recommend natural wooden or ceramic combs. Brushes with natural bristles can be a good choice. The scales are smoother and hair is shiny after using them. A brush must be coated with an antistatic agent.

Combing. Combing. Start at the ends and work your way to the root.

If you do not have blood pressure problems, you can comb your locks with your head tilted. This will allow blood to flow to the head and reach the roots.

You should buy two combs if you have long hair. A comb with thicker teeth and a massage brush. You can now safely untangle hair from the root to the ends by using a comb.

If your hair is short (less than shoulder length), you can start comb immediately at the roots and continue along the length. You won't get as messy with a short haircut. If you do keep your hair long, trim the ends often. Avoid injury to your scalp by choosing a brush with a broad working surface that doesn't have sharp teeth.

Hair with curly curls needs special attention. We have very few teeth for special combs that are designed to comb wavy hair. As with long hair, curls can be combed. This includes both short and long hair. Combs start by untangling the ends then move to the roots. You can use this type hair with only a comb made of rare teeth.

Chapter 16: Hair Loss Classification

There are several ways hair loss can be classified. First, examine the patient's scalp. This will help determine if hair is falling out due to damage to the hair follicles.

There are two types of hair loss: scarring and non-scarring. A healthy scalp indicates that there is no scarring. It seems unoccupied because it has lots of follicular architecture. Scarring of hair loss can be a sign that something is wrong with the follicles.

No matter whether there's scarring on the scalp or not, you will see areas of visible hair loss. A biopsy is performed on the scalp to determine the condition. In some cases, doctors will pull hairs in order to assess the condition. These types are available for both scarring and unscarring hair loss.

Non-scarring hair loss

Alopecia Areata

Alopecia Areata is a common type of baldness. It typically starts as a quarter-sized, smooth baldness. It usually regrows within three to six months with no treatment. Sometimes, hair grows back in places where it was dark before.

Alopecia totalis, a severe type of this alopecia, is a form that can be extended. In this situation, the entire scalp is bald. You should note, however, that hair loss in specific areas (such as bald spots) is not a widespread condition.

Alopecia also can affect other parts. The most common condition is the loss of eyebrows.

Stress has been linked with Alopecia Areata. Some people believe hair loss is caused by stress. However, some studies prove the reverse. The patient suffering from alopecia experiences stress. This condition is known as an autoimmune disorder. It attacks its own hair follicles and causes hair loss.

The bald areas are treated with small amounts of steroids. This stimulates faster hair growth. Oral steroids may also be available.

This can be disguised easily by simply combing. For those with more severe cases, a hairpiece can be used to cover it or to shave the entire head.

Traction Alopecia

Traction alopecia, or hair loss that occurs in one area of the body, is caused when hair is pulled repeatedly. This condition is common among people who have tight hairstyles and a ponytail. Their hair eventually falls out due to their tight hairstyles.

Trichotillomania

Trichotillomania can be described as the voluntary practice or inclination to pull one's own hair. The eyelashes are most often affected by this condition. The patches of affected eyelashes are usually smooth and free from evidences such as broken-off hairs. This is not like other forms. Treatment depends on the individual's behavior. The solution is to become aware of the habits they have and stop doing them. Some cases are due to anxiety.

Tinea Capitis

Tinea can be a medical term that refers a fungal infection. Capitis is a synonym for head. It is a medical condition in the which hair loss can be caused by fungal infection on scalp. The areas that are bald often have broken hairs. Patients can also use oral antifungals, which penetrate the hair roots to cure the infection. This is to aid hair growth. You can avoid this by not borrowing hair brushes and/or combs.

Generalized Hair loss

The generalized loss of hair does not indicate balding patterns. This is a general hair thinning that can be felt when the hair feels dry. It could be telogen efluvium (the hair loss after childbirth, physical stress), androgenetic, or androgenetic (male and female pattern baldness).

Scarring Hair Loss

Scarring is a common hair loss condition. It usually affects about 3%. Although rare, it can sometimes be a sign of an internal condition.

While this is uncommon, scarring hair may result in permanent and irreversible loss. Sometimes scarring hair loss begins with tiny patches that grow over time. Others are more gradual and less noticeable. Scarring hair loss due to scarring can happen quickly.

Scarring alopecia patches may have rough edges. Because the condition typically begins in the scalp, there will be no noticeable baldness around the affected area. In rare cases, redness may be present.

These can help diagnose scarring, but sometimes biopsies will still be required.

Inflammation of cells around the hair follicles can lead to scarring. It leads to the destruction and formation of scar tissue. As the disease spreads, it causes pain. This can cause permanent damage to hair follicles, and eventually hair loss.

The hair loss will stop after the alopecia reaches the stage of burnt-out. Either the bald areas can be surgically removed, or they can be planted with hair follicles taken from unaffected regions.

THE BASICS OF HAIR LOSS: HOW HAIR GREENS

Hair is comprised of a protein known as Keratin. In terms of the way in which hair is laid out it is evident when looking at it closely that it is divided into three layers: an outer cuticle and middle cortex, and a the central medulla. The three layers are the way that hair is arranged on your head. these layers could contribute to the hair loss you could be experiencing.

Hair is produced from a follicle. This is the tiny hole or space in your head that hair is pushed out of.Many occasions, when people suffer from hair loss it could be due to the follicles have become blocked and the new hairs don't have a method of reaching the surface. This is typically one of the causes that contribute to loss of hair overall.

If you're losing hair it is possible to look into a solution for the hair follicles. It's a possibility that this will not cause loss of hair but if you're suffering from thin hair, getting a couple of the follicles disconnected and permitting new hairs to develop is something you can try.

If you're not planning to lose all your hair when you reach an age group, you might be able to defer this for a bit by making the effort to do something to your hair follicles.

There are a variety of locations where you can get shampoos, as well as other items that can help you unblock your hair follicles. If you are able to locate things that you can use and start with a treatment plan and follow the steps, you will notice that your hair is coming in faster and that you could have more than you imagined previously.

But these procedures must be continued, so make sure to follow instructions to ensure that you're doing all you can to achieve the most hair you can get.

Be aware that once you've begun to use specific shampoos to help wash the hair follicles of your scalp You will need to keep using these shampoos as if do not, you're likely to notice that the hair won't be growing at the rate you'd prefer it to.

Keep this in mind as a thing to be aware of prior to starting the hair regrowth treatment.Most of these treatments will have to continue going for a long time therefore, if this is something important to you, then you must begin with the goal of keeping track of them.

Understanding the Growth Cycle

The process of growing hair is different for humans than for other animals anywhere in the world. If you own pets, or don't, you're likely to know that in certain seasons their hair grows extremely long and thick, while in other seasons, they shed excessively. Animals shed their hair in this way

biologically physically always indoors and not exposed to any change

seasons. Humans however are not shedding with predictable frequency. Hair remains a component of

A cycle, similar to the hair of animals however, each hair on our heads is in a different stage of the cycle.

So, our hair is always growing and shedding at the same time. It's common to shed between 25 and 100 hairs each day generally our hair grows around 6 inches

Every year, but this can occur with a flurry at times.

There are three phases to growing hair: catagen anagen, and telogen. The catagen stage lasts for about a year.

for up to three weeks , and causes hair to go through an era of transition. The hair is stopped growing

The outer root then is able to shrink in order to fight the root in the hair follicle. This is referred to as a

club hair.

The next stage is the telogen stage. Hair is more likely to fall out in this stage since hair is in rest. The hair then transitions to the anagen stage. This is the active phase of hair growth, and hair grows quickly. The anagen stage lasts between two and six years. So if your hair appears to grow extremely slowly, then you may have a shorter anagen phase.

It is common for baldness to occur when hair loses its hair at the telogen stage, and it is then unable to regenerate.

This could be due to a variety of reasons. For instance, if your hair follicle has become blocked and hair is not pushing

Through and the root dies. If hair falls out, most of the time it will regrow, however, if it does not

Renew itself and the root diesand will never.

Common Causes of Hair Loss

There are many who believe that loss of hair is caused by a disease or that it is the result of an illness.

But, it's not the case. The majority of cases of baldness are due to a medical condition or illness, but it can be caused by a combination of both.

It is typically a result of the influence of a variety of aspects. The causes could include the effects of aging, heredity and

the levels of testosterone throughout your body. They are the main reason for the typical patterns for both genders.

the baldness that is discovered. But, there are many other reasons that could be causing

the loss of your hair or contributes to the loss of your hair, or contributing significantly to.

One of the reasons can be hormonal imbalances. This could mean everything from thyroid issues to

childbirth, or perhaps taking birth control pills. An illness of serious nature could cause loss of

hair loss - for example, an ovarian tumor and adrenal glands or an illness such as a fever. Certain medicines,

Like chemotherapy for cancer, can cause hair loss out, but only after you stop taking these medications, it will be gone.

If you take medication that treat hair loss, it will typically be able to grow back.

There are other triggers that could be causing you to get sick and they could be as simple as shampooing your hair.

hair too frequently or blow drying it excessively. In many instances like those, people were more at risk of

hair loss pattern however, as they continued to wash their hair or blow dry their hair too frequently the hair loss became more severe.

They were losing more hair, and were losing hair more rapidly.

Other causes could be physical or emotional stress. This can result in loss of hair. Additionally, the nervous habits one might be prone to, such as pulling hair out or rubbing their scalp, and other factors, could result in hair loss. The effects of radiation therapy, burns and ringworm can also be the cause for loss of hair. loss.Most of these reasons don't cause hair loss by themselves. However, one will be more prone to lose their hair if they suffer from one or more of these issues and also experience the family's history of losing hair.

If you are a member of your family and you're aware that you're prone to balding pattern and loss of hair, you must be certain to take take care of the hair. Don't engage in any activity which could lead to or cause an increase in hair loss. There may not be any way that you can do to stop the loss of your hair however you can take steps to lessen the severity or last until you're older.

STRIKING A BALANCE What causes the imbalance?

Your hair can reveal a amount about you, and that includes the condition the body you are wearing is balance. Balance is having good mental and physical health, and being the ability to fully

functioning glands and organs that produce the proper hormones needed by your body. If there is a

If someone is physically and mentally hair will to be much healthier.

Shiny and beautiful, their scalp will be healthy and soft and moist. Hair will be

They can tell you many things about their overall health status is, both in terms of mental and physical

health.

If a person isn't well, whether physically well, or mentally well their hair is likely to be

A bit dull, and they're likely to have a difficult to focus on what their hair ought to look rather dull and boring. The hair is dull and boring.

If you are a person who is unhealthy If you're a person who's unhealthy, you'll be able to notice periods where their hair falls out. It

could become waxy due to the excess production of glands making your hair

nutrients.

It's also a proven fact that any change we are experiencing within our own lives is bound to

visible to all our heads. If we're well-being and happy our heads will reflect that.

this. If we don't, our hair may be falling out, and there could be an ebb in mental or physical state

is easily visible in hair.

Although excitement and challenge is a requirement to stay attractive and active

For some people, stress can cause hair to fall off from our head. When this happens

It will generally grow it is possible to keep our bodies in order and go through the stressors without being able to fall back into them.

Keep this in mind if you're losing hair due to stress or losing hair due to a

no matter what stage of your life, you're really in the right place to be in regards to your hair.

loss because, it is the case that after you have fixed what's happening in your life the hair will grow back

The hair will grow and the loss can be reversed. Therefore, if you've lost hair because of stress or

To be mentally or physically in a state of mental or physical illness, the good news is that when you are your health back and are healthy, you will be back

On the right track, you're not going to need to worry about your hair. It will grow back in its own way.

BLACK HAIR BASICS

The normal hair and hair follicles of people of African descent are tightly curled, thereby creating hair that curls. Black hair is also generally has a greater in diameter than Caucasian hair, and it retains less water, resulting in its comparative "kinkiness." Hair of African descent is prone to kinkiness. numerous styles that are applied to Black hair may cause hair loss.

Black hair is extremely strong, and that's so since Black hairstyles put an immense amount of strain on the hair and scalp.For instance using a hairpick to lift hair into a bushy cut is extremely effective.

The process is damaging due to the continuous pulling that puts strain on hair's shaft and the hair follicle. In reality combing Black hair generally causes stress to Black hair, causing breaks, which can lead to dryness.

Cornrows and braids are two methods of hairstyling that pull hair in a tighter position, and this could cause a lot of stress to the scalp and hair, which can result in loss of hair. Braiding that leads to hair being pulled tightly can result in trauma alopecia, which is a loss of hair that is caused by injury of the hair as well as the scalp.Traumatic Alopecia can be reversed by taking care of your hair.

Relaxers and hot combs used to straighten hair can result in an abundance of heat and harm to the scalp and hair as well as result in traumatic alopecia, and, over time, can lead to permanent loss of hair. This is particularly true when processing of hair chemically is pulled tightly by rollers or high-temperature curling iron.

Conditioners made of hot oils are great for Black hair because the hot oil treatments are rich in polymers and proteins essential for fixing the cuticles of the hair. Hot oil treatments require heating the oil, then applying it to the scalp and hair after which hair is covered with a plastic cap in order to let the oil absorb.

Be sure to follow the guidelines for the treatment you're using to determine the amount of time you need to allow the treatment to be applied to the hair. The process will heal broken hair and more shinier hair will result.

Take into consideration that the hair relaxers typically employed on Black hair are made up of the chemical lye, or similar ones which break down hair shaft. If left on for longer than the recommended amount of time for use, these chemicals could consume the hair, causing the hair's clumps to split. This is why the same substances are found in products such as Drano(r) to clear the drains that have become blocked by hair.

Relaxers with no lye are very well-known today, mostly because they make people think that it isn't caustic. However, this is not the reality. The calcium hydroxide and carbonate of guanidine are made into guanidine hydroxide that can just as easily wash the water in a sink. The repeated use of these products may cause some hair loss. And if the scalp is damaged by these chemicals, hair loss could be permanent on that part of the scalp.

It is important to ask yourself if it appropriate to apply chemical toxins in hair regularly to achieve a desired appearance? This question should be addressed by every individual, but the facts must be clear.

There's not much which can be accomplished to stop this issue without changing the hairstyles that are typical for African Americans. There's a catch-22 when it comes to relaxing Black hairbecause brushing natural Black hair is a source of stress and breaks to hair and chemicals can cause much damage to scalp and hair as well.

There are several hair-relaxing products available which use chemicals, and are less aggressive as sodium hydroxide (lye) or its well-known counterpart for "no-lye" relaxers calcium hydroxide (quicklime) combined with carbonate of guanidine. One of them is Natural-Laxer(r)and Sahara Clay(r) by Baka ProductsTM, which has been available since the year 1990.

The product is completely natural and is not a lot of the harmful chemicals that are found in

commercial relaxers, and in reality contains only a finely ground herb known as Daphne Gnidium, and clay (from Africa it is believed to be quite secure. It is true that this product will do not smooth hair the majority of cases in the same manner as commercial relaxers, but it can increase the flexibility of Black hair less manageable.

There's another product that claims to be between 92 and 96% organic. It is known as Naturalaxer Kit in A Jar(tm)that doesn't require that the user brush through hair before applying it and causes less damage.

Of course, the main point is that If you are able to let your hair be as it is, you'll experience less stress and less damage to your hair, and therefore reduce at the very least one of the causes of loss of hair. The trend is growing for a portion of the Black populace that is getting more comfortable wearing their hair in natural , unstyled styles. One of these styles is the dreadlocks. There are a lot of stories and myths about the dreadlocks style, since there's no information of a proper quality available about this particular style like with all things that is misunderstood , many myths are created in the context of the style.

Dreadlocks should be cleaned; otherwise, they'll stink like all other hair that is dirty. The best method for washing dreadlocks is utilize a non-residue-free shampoo. The majority of commercially-made shampoos leave a residue, and may cause hair to not lock in the first place, thereby fueling the notion that hair needs become dirty before it could form hair dreadlocks. Clean hair actually locks better than hair that is dirty, because dirt can leave an in-and-of-itself residue which prevents locks from being formed.

To get the best results, make use of a fragrance-free shampoo with no conditioner. Dreadlocks are not tolerant to oils and greasy substances, however there are many great products available currently that can assist in creating Dreadlocks.

Dreadlocks are created by a process, and not just by brushing or combing the hair.

In general, it is recommended to start with hair around two inches long, and hair should be divided into squares that are even and then twisted in a gentle manner with a bonding or gel substance. A lot of people use natural beeswax that has none petroleum, whereas others utilize twist and loc gels specially designed specifically for locks.

When hair is separated and bent into small locks, it's important to leave them alone and allow to naturally bond. The amount of time required to form locks will be contingent on the thickness of your hair, however you can expect to wait a few months before the locks begin to develop.

When hair locks and locking, it must be cleaned. This is why washing needs to be prolonged for a time in order that hair is left to lock for about two weeks or one month.

Without manipulation.

If you do clean your hair you should use an elastic cap, or "do-rag" with low-pressure water to ensure that your newly formed locks aren't loosened. It is necessary to rinse for a longer amount of time than you usually dodue to the less pressure in the water, and also the lack of the direct control of the hair using your hands.

The water is beneficial for hair and locks process, which isn't a problem. It is essential that you make use of shampoos that do not include a conditioner and leaves the least amount of residue. A tiny amount of research is required here and your local health food store should have several natural shampoos. A skilled professional or a person you trust to re-twist the hair with a gentle touch, applying the gel for twisting or beeswax that you have used before.

Repeat this procedure every two weeks or one month. The more time you can be patient, the better. Eventually, in a matter of months, you will notice your hair beginning to form locks. Also, if you've got hair of a fine quality instead of a kinky type of hair hairdresser who is skilled in forming locks ("locktician") or a person who is knowledgeable about the hairstyle must be sought out.

While dreadlocks are generally the hairstyle of Blacks but there are many other races who enjoy the hairstyle. It is generally thought to be a kind of hair which, in the long run, can give your scalp and hair a break from the stress of heat and chemical treatments, as well as intense brushing and combing and consequently, can provide longer-lasting hair.

Skin Cancer: A RISK SURVEYOR OF LOSS OF HAIR

If you're losing your hair, your primary problem might not be coping with the shameful hair loss. There are real health risks associated with this condition since your head is normally covered with hair. One of the risks is melanoma or skin cancer.

Skin cancer, if not treated, can grow all over your body, and, eventually, end up killing you. If you have skin cancer, you should seek treatment.

If you are losing your hair or are losing your hair, it is vital to take preventative measures to lower your chance of contracting skin cancer.

Skin cancer is caused by the sun in the majority of instances. The skin that covers the upper part of the head isn't meant to be used to be used for

exposure to sunshine, your skin is particularly vulnerable to sun exposure. There are a lot of steps to ease your

skin when you are in the skin in the sun. These apply to more than just on your scalp, but your skin

everywhere.

The first step is to invest in a top-quality sunscreen. Choose an oil or spray that comes from an established brand to ensure the product is of good quality. The sunscreen you choose to use can be spray or lotion however, it should have at least SPF15. Check the instructions in the label and apply the directions, applying it as often as suggested. Make sure that the sunscreen you are using is water-resistant or not. If you plan to swim or sweat often, you should use sunscreen that is waterproof.

It is also recommended to wear protective clothing to protect yourself from skin cancer. Find hats that are lightweight or even over

Covers for the head to stop the sun's rays from getting to the skin. Sunglasses are essential to shield your skin

your eyes. It is particularly important to wear protective clothes between the hours of 10 am and 2 pm, in the time of

in the summer, during which it is the time when sun's at its highest. Be sure to take precautions

in winter, too. Even though the air isn't warm doesn't mean the sun's rays will not be

It is not harmful. In the sun-filled days of winter months, you should protect your skin by wearing clothing and sunscreen, as well as

You would do it during the summer.

Finally, avoid using tanning beds or other tanning devices, or relaxing in the sun to

a tan. Utilizing tanning oils is specifically detrimental to the skin. They may look attractive but the dangers are not

is worth is worth it. It is worth it. removed surgically in the very beginning stages of it and, therefore, it is advisable to choose

Participation in sports is a risky activity under the sun. You might end up getting cancer. Be aware

methods to stop it steps to prevent it, particularly if you're suffering from hair loss or hair loss that is causing it.

is not designed for exposure to the sun.

In the past all you could do if lost your hair was to buy an hat and

Learn to accept your appearance. There are many alternatives to

to treat hair loss. And there are other treatments you've never thought of. It is possible to

Choose to suffer with the loss of hair You can also consider alternatives to consider.

If you've made the decision to address the loss of your hair there are many things you need to be doing.

The most important thing you can do is talk about your concerns with someone whom you feel comfortable, such as your doctor.

The first thing to remember is that talking to your physician is crucial since he may be

You can get recommendations for things you've never ever heard of. If the doctor knows the medical background of you, he will be

you will discover that you're much more successful if you have him have a look and look at what he sees

is to look around the possibilities, and suggest suggestions to you.

At present, there are two approved medically to combat hair loss. These medications

It has been discovered that they can reduce hair loss. The most common drugs used are drugs for high blood pressure are known to stop hair loss.

Have had negative side effects that include disappearance of the hair loss among those who

They eventually took the pills. After that the hair loss medications were developed. They have been used for a short time with minimal results.

The results of stopping hair loss, however, before you start taking these supplements, you must consult your

Doctor to ensure that you are using them safely for use by you.

If you're not ready to get prescribed medication for lost hair, then there's many non-medical options

which could cause hair growth which could grow your hair back. Although they haven't been approved by the FDA that could cause hair loss, they are there

Evidence suggests that they can cause hair growth. If you're interested in this to learn more, consult your doctor, then conduct some study to find out what kind of treatments will work best for you. Be aware that there are laser treatments that can be applied to your head, which can cause hair growth or at the very least stop the loss of hair.

Keep in mind that in these situations there is evidence that it is effective in certain people however it is not effective on other people. Due to this, it is crucial to talk with your physician prior to start any of these procedures or tests.

SCALP AND HAIR DISEASES

There are many scalp and hair diseases. Some are quite frequent, while some more serious scalp and hair conditions are extremely rare.

Alopecia Areata is an autoimmune skin condition that triggers the immune system of the body to attack hair follicles that cause hair loss in patches. It can affect 1.7

per cent of world's population, with 4.7 million people living in the United States.

If the condition gets to the point that all hair on the scalp is gone this is known as Alopecia Totalis, and where hair loss extends to the entire body, it's known as Alopecia Universialis. There isn't a known cause of alopecia areata and consequently no known cure. It usually begins to manifest at the age of 20 and does not appear to favor one race or gender.

Alopecia areata is alopecia that occurs in phases which sees hair growing back but falling out of a series of phases. Seborrheic Dermatitis, which is a severe type of seborrhea is a non-infectious skin disease that can cause excessive oiliness of the skin mostly on the scalp. This is due to the overproduction of sebum the substance that is produced by the body in order to lubricate the area where hair follicles reside.

Seborrhea is the condition where oiliness occurs without scaling or redness. The condition is typically seen in middle-aged, infants and those over 65, and is often referred to in infants as the cradle cap. There is no cure for the disease but in infants it typically disappears over the course of. In adults, the condition can remain with different levels of severity. Redness, swelling and flaking frequently are signs of this condition.

It can be treated easily with the use of creams with corticosteroids, as well as shampoos that contain pine tar, salicylic acid, or selenium sulfur.

Seborrhea and seborrheic Dermatitis can be managed and treated, and is important to treat them as if left untreated they could contribute to loss of hair. In reality, a group consisting of Japanese Scientists have linked the excess production of sebum to loss of hair. The reason for this is that sebaceous glands located in the areas of the scalp that are where hair loss is occurring or where there is no hair are larger, which are believed to trigger the obstruction of pores as well as numerous other conditions that cause hair loss.

Psoriasis is known as an immune-mediated condition that affects various parts as well as functions in the human body. It isn't contagious, as one of the regions of the body that it may be affecting includes the hair. It is typically seen as red patches on the skin that is accompanied by burning or itching. There are a variety of factors thought to trigger the development of psoriasis. Some of them are the stress of emotional trauma, some infections, toxemia, thinning of the intestinal wall and the adverse reactions to certain medications.

About half of those with psoriasis suffer from scalp psoriasis. Like seborrheaand scalp psoriasis, scalp p is a condition that if not treated can lead to hair loss.

Fortunately, it is able to be treated using a range of creams and shampoos with salicylic acid and tar. It is essential to avoid scratching the scalp or pick at the scabs the condition causes, as it could cause damage to the dermis hair follicles and lead to permanent loss of hair. For as long as

hair follicles aren't damaged, the loss of hair that is due to this condition is usually short-lived and hair will regrow after the condition is gone. The most effective ways to alleviate itching is making use of household products like mouthwashes, such as Lavoris(r) or Listerine(r). Carbolated Vaseline(r) can be used on the hairline to alleviate the symptoms.

Hair dyes of every kind and chemical treatments like relaxers and permanents should avoid at all cost for those suffering from Psoriasis. They are very harmful overall however, they can be harmful in particular.

Psoriasis sufferers can cause irreparable destruction of the hair follicle in the course of a short time.

As with all of these illnesses, one should be aware that psoriasis can't be treated with drugs. If there is a cure, it will be through the body repairing itself by the correcting of any malfunctions within the body.

A common condition that affects all sufferers of psoriasis is toxemia. When the body is toxic, a variety of genetic dispositions develop and psoriasis is just one of the ailments that is because of the condition known as toxemia.

Toxemia is caused due to poor circulation and thinning of intestinal wall. The patient's blood is acidic, and the acidity is absorbed through the biggest organ in the body, the skin. Psoriasis sufferers have been treated with natural procedures like cleansing the body internally, avoiding alcohol, increasing consumption of water, particularly distillation water and exposure to sunlight in certain instances, the reduction of stress through the elimination of the stress

conditions, and practicing meditation and the elimination of nighthades like tobacco, tomatoes white potatoes, eggplant, peppers (not black pepper) and the spice paprika.

One food that can be common to people suffering from psoriasis, is pizza. Naturally, it is made up of tomatoes. Pizza also has every ingredient that an individual suffering from psoriasis should stay clear of including the white flour and peppers,, and hot spices. Pizza is also highly acidic and must be absconding from by all means.

Alongside the dietary tips mentioned earlier it is recommended that people suffering from psoriasis eat lamb, fish and poultry regularly, eat an alkaline diet, and drink buttermilk or milk with a low fat content. Fish, in particular canned or fresh salmon, sardines, and albacore tuna in its white form, contains Omega-3 fatty acids, which are essential for scalp and skin health. While most fish are advised avoid dark-fleshed species like bluefish and mackerel sushi, or shellfish.

Poultry like cornishhens, turkey, chicken and other fowls that aren't fat are great for people who suffer from psoriasis if they are not fried.To keep away from excess fat take off the skin prior to eating and avoid fowl which is high in fat like duck and goose. Lamb is the sole recommended red meat for people suffering from psoriasis. This is due to the fact that it is simple to digest, and still an excellent food source for protein. It should, of course, be cooked in any way, except for frying.

The consumption of dairy products must be with care and should be consumed only in low-fat or nonfat dairy products are recommended for people suffering from psoriasis may get calcium from the sources mentioned in the earlier section on Diet, Nutrition and Hair Loss like celery, soybean products as well as lettuce and greens.

White bread is a bad idea to avoid. Also, a small portion of whole grain bread as well as whole grain products may be substituted but should be consumed with care because all grains, except millet, contain acid-forming. In addition, it is best to stop all alcohol consumption, with the exception for maybe small glasses of red wine after dinner to boost blood circulation and digestive health.

Lecithin can be beneficial to psoriasis sufferers It can be taken in granular form at the amount of 1 teaspoon three times daily every day, seven days per week, whether plain or mixed with water or juice, sprinkled over cereal or salad. When the condition has gone away decrease the dosage to one tablespoon once every day, for five days per week.

Lecithin is available in every health store and even though it can be purchased in tablet or liquid form, as well as in its granular form, it's preferred to be consumed in granular form due to its large amount of phosphatide in it when consumed in this manner. The doses recommended should not be exceeding, since the excessive consumption of lecithin may result in a blockage of the calcium absorption.

Eczema is yet another non-infectious skin condition that resembles the psoriasis condition very closely.Eczema results in scales, reddened inflamed skin that occasionally releases pus, and the well-known itching that is a major discomfort to people suffering from it. They are, however, two distinct conditions that require different treatment.

There are a few remedies on psoriasis, and they work for Eczema as well. Eczema can cause massive buildup of pus and scalp sores and may cause extreme scarring. The accumulation caused by eczema may cause temporary loss of hair however , the scarring that could result from scratching the painfully itchy lesions could result in permanent harm to hair follicles.

Eczema is a condition caused by toxemia , too. While one may make use of the many medications and creams available that are available to treat its symptoms, permanent relief is likely to be achieved by removing the underlying cause for the toxemia.

Cleaning and drinking plenty of clean water are the best way to fight Eczema. The majority of the nutritional suggestions are the same for those suffering with eczema. However, there's usually an increase in susceptibility to fish, so it is recommended that it be consumed in a small quantity. In addition, there is generally an extremely high level of intolerance to dairy products, as eczema is a common cause of allergies. This is why it is suggested to make use of goat's or soy milk instead.

Hair loss as a result of chemotherapy is a typical result of treatment. Chemotherapy kills cancerous cells that reproduce quickly. cells, but the negative consequence of chemotherapy is that it also destroys rapidly reproducing cells that stimulate hair growth and nails.

Hair loss is rapid and in large amounts generally. In this time it is not possible to find prescription or herbal prescription-only treatment of any type has been discovered to help maintain the hair. Fortunately, hair usually is restored within six months to one year after treatment stops.

Patients have noticed that hair grown after chemotherapy is finer with texture, and has a lighter color initially. This is usually a temporary condition that get better with time.

Patients recovering from chemotherapy should stay clear of chemical treatments like perms, relaxers bleaching and coloring the hair until it has grown at least 3 inches, and not before a minimum of one year after the final treatment. Chemotherapy can trigger skin sensitivities and the chemicals may cause extreme irritation on the scalp.

DIET, NUTRITION , AND HAIR LOSS

The most important factor to maintain the growth of protein in the biological body is that it is essential to maintain a healthy diet. Although some factors have been proven to be factors that cause hair loss, it is important to remember that hair is a part of the entire biological system of the human body.

v/pod-product-compliance